SpringerBriefs in Molecular Science

Chemistry of Foods

Series editor

Salvatore Parisi, Industrial Consultant, Palermo, Italy

More information about this series at http://www.springer.com/series/11853

Luciano Piergiovanni · Sara Limbo

Food Packaging Materials

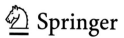 Springer

Luciano Piergiovanni
Department of Food, Environmental and
  Nutritional Sciences (DeFENS)
Università degli Studi di Milano
Milan
Italy

Sara Limbo
Department of Food, Environmental and
  Nutritional Sciences (DeFENS)
Università degli Studi di Milano
Milan
Italy

ISSN 2191-5407   ISSN 2191-5415   (electronic)
SpringerBriefs in Molecular Science
ISSN 2199-689X   ISSN 2199-7209   (electronic)
Chemistry of Foods
ISBN 978-3-319-24730-4   ISBN 978-3-319-24732-8   (eBook)
DOI 10.1007/978-3-319-24732-8

Library of Congress Control Number: 2015952044

Springer Cham Heidelberg New York Dordrecht London

Springer International Publishing AG Switzerland is part of Springer Science+Business Media
(www.springer.com)

Contents

Chapter 1
Introduction to Food Packaging Materials

Abstract Basically, Packaging Science is Materials Science. As a consequence, the right choice of a package largely depends on the performance of the packaging materials used. These performances may be expressed in a chemical and physical way. On the other hand, a technical description in terms of material chemistry can be useful. This book introduces the chemical peculiarities of four different material categories: plastics, cellulosic, ceramic and metals. Nevertheless, a large variability of different items are obtained in these four categories by means of even small chemical changes. Moreover, important changes in the final properties and performances of food packaging materials can be obtained by means of chemical modifications. Finally, the current situation of food packaging materials is briefly described in terms of global amount of unit sales worldwide.

Keywords Cellulosic materials · Ceramic materials · Food packaging materials · Metals · Packaging science · Plastic materials · World packaging consumption

Abbreviations

WPO   World Packaging Organisation

1.1   Foreword

This brief is concerned with the material chemistry of food packaging materials. It introduces the properties and peculiarities of typical packaging materials. Packaging Science, to a large extent, is Materials Science, i.e. the right choice of a package largely depends on the performance of the packaging materials used. These performances are related to both their chemical and physical properties but can be mainly explained and described in terms of material chemistry. Materials used to pack foods are plastics, cellulosic, ceramic, and metals. Nevertheless, a large variability of different items are obtained in these four categories by means of even small chemical changes. Therefore, the book introduces chemical peculiarities of

© The Author(s) 2016
L. Piergiovanni and S. Limbo, *Food Packaging Materials*,
Chemistry of Foods, DOI 10.1007/978-3-319-24732-8_1

these four materials. In addition, it also describes how it is possible to achieve important changes in the final properties and performances by means of chemical modifications in the structure and in the composition.

Moreover, some possible peculiar reactions between materials components and food ingredients (or environmental constituents) are also very important when speaking of packaging and food packaging in particular. These reactions can reduce the performance of packages, affecting also the recycling processes, influencing the product quality and much more. The last part of the book is therefore related to metal corrosion, chemical resistance and degradability phenomena of the main packaging materials.

1.2 Facts and Figures

Huge amount of materials are used worldwide to produce packaging materials and packages: more than two thirds are used by the food sector. This amount is continuously increasing because of changes occurring in habits of food preparation and consumption, as well as the positive development of various areas and markets in the world (Iascone et al. 2014; McCloskey 2012; Vercesi 2008) where packaging still has a large opportunity of increase. In detail, according to recent researches (Iascone et al. 2014):

- The Asia and Pacific region has the highest number of used packages between 2011 and 2013 (15.2 %; 1,869,856 used packages in 2013)
- The European Union, North America and the South-American Area are distant enough (6.0, 4.4 and 3.5 %, respectively)
- The Eastern Europe can reach 2.9 % of the total number of used packages on condition that Russian data are added
- Central Asia and the African continent can reach only 1.2 %, while the lowest result is ascribed to Australia and New Zealand (aggregate result: 0.3 %; 37,687 used packages in 2013).

The global amount of packaging sales are estimated to account for $797 billion in 2013 but are expected to grow at an annual rate of 4 % to 2018. Obviously, the growth of packaging sector is drawing a special attention to recycling opportunities and processes which are in a strong relationship with materials chemistry and composition and Fig. 1.1 shows the market share of different packaging materials (Wood 2012; WPO 2008). Glass and metals, despite their share, due to their density which is at least three times the ones of paper and plastics, undoubtedly are the most abundant materials used for packaging as far as the mass of materials, not the number of packages, is concerned.

Actually, the lightest packaging materials such as paper and board, plastic and composites definitely represent the most relevant sector for food packaging at present. In addition, this field of production processes is the one where it is possible to recognise the foremost variability of kinds and constituents.

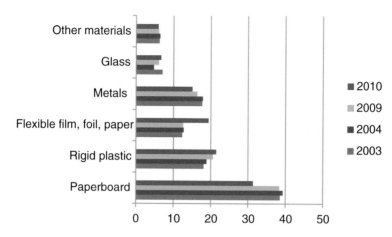

Fig. 1.1 The percentage of market share of different packaging materials used in packaging between 2003 and 2010 (Wood 2012; WPO 2008)

References

Iascone B, Iascone P, Aldrigo D (2014) Market data, Imballaggio in cifre 2014. In: Iascone B, Iascone P, Aldrigo D (eds) Imballaggio in cifre, vol 2014. The Italian Institute of Packaging, Milan

McCloskey M (2012) Globalization, health and the nutrition transition: how Global TNCs are changing local food consumption patterns. Dissertation, University of Puget Sound. http://soundideas.pugetsound.edu/cgi/viewcontent.cgi?article=1005&context=ipe_theses. Accessed 21 May 2015

Vercesi S (2008) Market dynamics in the food industry. A new logic to sustain value creation. Dissertation, Copenhagen Business School. http://studenttheses.cbs.dk/bitstream/handle/10417/357/stefania_vercesi.pdf?sequence=1. Accessed 21 May 2015

Wood B (2012) Packaging outpaces overall economy. Plast Technol. http://www.ptonline.com/columns/packaging-outpaces-overall-economy. Accessed 05 June 2015

WPO (2008) Market statistics and future trends in global packaging. WPO—World Packaging Organisation/PIRA International Ltd.), World Packaging Organisation. http://www.worldpackaging.org

Chapter 2
Ceramic Packaging Materials

Abstract The term 'ceramic' refers to a category of materials that can be all defined as inorganic and non-metallic, and whose chemistry is mainly based on silicon structures. Substantially, these products are subdivided in two categories, depending on the main component: glass on the one hand, and minor ceramic materials like china, porcelain and earthenware on the other side. Common glasses can have different chemical composition, leading to their own colour, thermal or mechanical resistance. Silicon, commonly represented as silica, is found as silica or silicates. With relation to the crystalline structure, silicon's four valences lead to a structural unit in which each silicon atom is located at the centre of a tetrahedron. For this reason, crystalline structures are typical and commonly found in all silicon-based ores. Glass packages are well known because of their optical, thermal and mechanical properties. On the other side, non-glass packages are commonly subdivided in two subgroups: porous earthenware and non-porous porcelain. Each different sub-type shows peculiar properties with notable importance when speaking of food packaging applications.

Keywords Ceramic · Glass · Non-porous porcelain · Porous earthenware · Glass physical properties · Ultraviolet transmission coefficient

Abbreviations

SiO_2 Silicon dioxide
UV   Ultraviolet

2.1   Ceramic Packaging Materials: An Overview

In this section, the term 'ceramic' refers to a category of materials that can be all defined as inorganic and non-metallic, and whose chemistry is mainly based on silicon structures. Some minor ceramic materials like china, porcelain and earthenware are also used for the production of containers. However, less relevance

© The Author(s) 2016
L. Piergiovanni and S. Limbo, *Food Packaging Materials*,
Chemistry of Foods, DOI 10.1007/978-3-319-24732-8_2

will be reserved to these products being glass the most important and used material for packaging purposes. Ceramic containers are used for a wide variety of liquid, solid and semisolid foods, but the main use is typically for liquids and the bottle is the most common shape used. However, cups, jars, bowls, vases, amphora, as well as big containers such as tanks, reservoirs, cisterns and vessels are also made by ceramic materials and can get in contact with foods and beverages.

2.1.1   Glass

According to one of the most accurate and available definitions (ASTM 2010), glass is 'an amorphous, inorganic product of fusion that has been cooled to a rigid condition without crystallising'. In fact, the word glass applies more to a physical state of the matter than to a chemical structure; some special organic materials are also named 'glass' or 'glassy' (Mark et al. 1985).

Common glasses can have different chemical composition (Table 2.1), leading to their own colour, thermal or mechanical resistance. Anyway, the major component is always silicon (60–75 %), commonly represented as silica or silicon dioxide (SiO_2). Silicon is the most plentiful element on earth after oxygen; it is found as silica in quartz, sand, cristobalite, and many other minerals. In addition, silicon can be found as silicate—$[SiO_4]^{4-}$—in minerals such as feldspar and kaolinite, where silicon dioxide is joined to some metal oxides. With relation to the crystalline structure, the distinctive form of all silicon-based ores, silicon's four valences lead

Table 2.1 Chemical composition (expressed as %) of common glasses

	Soda-lime glass	Borosilicate glass	Amber	Green	Lead glass	Glass ceramics
Silica	71–73	65–85	72.6	72.1	60	40–70
Boron oxide	–	8–15	–	–	–	–
Sodium oxide	9–15	3–9	12.8	2.9	1.0	–
Potassium oxide	0–1.5	0–2	1.01	0.87	14.9	–
Calcium oxide	7–14	0–2.5	11.1	9.8	–	–
Magnesium oxide	0–6	–	0.23	1.74	–	10–30
Barium oxide	–	0–1	–	–	–	–
Lead oxide	–	–	–	–	24.0	–
Aluminum oxide	0–2	1–5	1.81	1.93	0.08	10–30
Mixture of iron (III) oxide and titanium dioxide	0–0.6	–	0.34	0.37	0.02	–
Chromium (III) oxide	–	–	0.002	0.17	–	–
Sulphur trioxide	–	–	0.08	0.09	–	–
Titanium dioxide	–	–	–	–	–	7–15

to a structural unit, in which each silicon atom is located at the centre of a tetrahedron, having four oxygen atoms at the corners (Fig. 2.1).

The tetrahedron arranges symmetrically and continuously, each oxygen being connected to two silicon atoms, leading to a well-ordered crystalline organisation. Silica shows a clear polymorphism being able to crystallise at different temperatures and leading to various forms available in the different ores (Demuth et al. 1999):

$$\alpha - \text{quartz} \overset{579°C}{\Leftrightarrow} \beta - \text{quartz} \overset{857°C}{\Leftrightarrow} \gamma - \text{tridymite} \overset{1,470°C}{\Leftrightarrow} \beta - \text{cristobalite} \quad (2.1)$$

The crystalline state of SiO_2 results in very high melting temperature, high toughness, low or null transparency and poor inertness. These features are opposite to expected characteristics of glass packages, when speaking of use and manufacture. Actually, the glass-making process changes inorganic ingredients (Table 2.2) from the crystalline to the amorphous state, through a mainly physical transformation which occurs at temperature above 1,450–1,500 °C. Crystalline structures are lost during this process and tetrahedral units reorganise in an amorphous structure (Fig. 2.2) including atoms of sodium, calcium and magnesium in empty spaces created by the rearrangement. Included metals come from minor ingredients of the

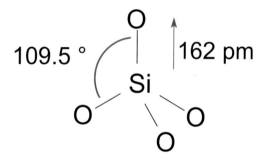

Fig. 2.1 With relation to crystalline form of silicon containing ores, each silicon atom is located at the centre of a tetrahedron, having four oxygen atoms at the corner. BKchem version 0.13.0, 2009 (http://bkchem.zirael.org/index.html) has been used for drawing this structure

Table 2.2 Ingredients used in the glass-making process and relative functions

Ingredient	Function
Silica sand	Former
Boron oxide	Former
Cullet (recycled glass)	Former, fluxes, energy saving
Sodium carbonate	Fluxes
Potassium carbonate	Fluxes
Calcium carbonate	Stabiliser
Magnesium carbonate	Stabiliser
Barium carbonate	Stabiliser
Sodium sulphate	Fining agent
Metal oxides	Colourant, bleaching

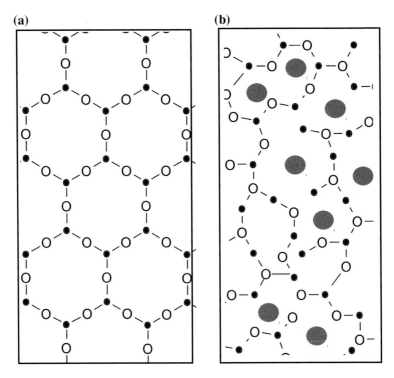

Fig. 2.2 A two-dimensional representation of the crystalline structure **a** (the *black circles* correspond to Silicon, the *clear* and *bigger circles* to Oxygena) of silicone containing ores and the amorphous one **b** (the *full grey biggest circles* to metals, such as sodium, calcium or magnesium) obtained after glass manufacture, which includes atoms of sodium, calcium and magnesium in the empty spaces

glass-making mixture (Lehman 2004; Nixon 2015) which are fundamental in establishing optical, thermal and mechanical properties of the final material (Table 2.3). The ability of the 'Si–O–Si' bond to display angles from 120 up to 180° (Chiang et al. 1997; Varshneya 1994; Rawson 1980) makes possible this amorphous, randomised structure and correlated main properties of glass containers.

2.1.1.1   Thermal Properties of Glass Packages

Glass is an amorphous material and it does not display a sharp melting temperature. In fact, it progressively softens until a true liquid state is achieved; subsequently, it becomes solid over a temperature range when cooling. In the most common glass used for packaging (a soda-lime glass based on a mixture of sodium carbonate and calcium carbonate), the higher the concentration of alkali, the lower the tetrahedral connectivity. This arrangement decreases the glass transition temperature (Chiang et al. 1997; Varshneya 1994) leading to lower temperatures of melting and

Table 2.3 Physical properties of soda lime versus borosilicate glasses (Lehman 2004; Nixon 2015)

Ingredient	Soda-lime glass	Borosilicate glass
Coefficient of linear expansion (°C^{-1}) α (0–300 °C)	8.6×10^{-6}	3.25×10^{-6}
Strain point (°C)	511	510
Annealing range (°C)	480–575	560
Soften point (°C)	575	821
Temperature limits (°C)		230 (normal service)
Maximum thermal shock (°C)		160
Density (g cm^{-3})	2.44	2.23
Young's modulus (GPa)	10.2	9.1
Shear modulus (modulus of rigidity) (GPa)	4.2	3.8
Refractive index (λ = 589.3 nm)	1.515	1.474

deformation, which are very useful behaviours for glass containers manufacture. Furthermore, glass melting and moulding can be indefinitely repeated without any loss of the original properties, giving great and unsurpassed opportunities of recycling to this material.

Glass has the lowest coefficient of thermal expansion among any packaging material (about 6–8 $\times$ 10^{-6} °C^{-1}). On the other side, this feature might augment the risk of failures when a glass container, closed with metal or plastic closures, undergoes to thermal treatment like pasteurisation or sterilisation. The most important thermal property of glass bottles or jars is the capability to withstand sudden thermal changes. Even if glass has low thermal conductivity (0.96 W m^{-1} °C^{-1} at 30 °C), a temperature variation deeply modifies the inner stress equilibrium. When glass is quickly cooled, tensile stresses are established on the surface from which the heat is removed first; tensile stresses are compensated by compressive stresses in the inner structure. On the contrary, when glass matrices are quickly heated, compressive forces are set up on the surface where its temperature increases first, with tensile forces on the opposite. Upon the temperature equilibrium is slowly achieved, however, these stresses disappear. Since glass is more sensitive to tensile stresses than to compressive ones, as many materials, sudden cooling steps are the most dangerous processes. The thermal strength of glass objects is influenced by the chemical composition; the presence of boron and aluminum oxides increases hugely the heat resistance (Table 2.3), like in Pyrex® or Corning® glasses respectively.

2.1.1.2 Mechanical Properties of Glass Packages

Glass containers are known as fragile objects: despite the high strength of the covalent bond between silicon and oxygen, an initiated fracture quickly propagates in glass items (Zhao et al. 2006). In fact, the continuous structure of interconnected tetrahedral SiO_2 can prevent plastic flows of the material; the same thing can be affirmed for stress absorption. Moreover, the breakage occurs when widely varying stresses are observed. Glass objects always have superficial or internal defects (cracks, flaws), even if not always visible, leading at their tip to a stress amplification. For these reasons glass bottles are tested for internal pressure resistance, vertical load strength and resistance to impact.

Vertical loads are quite common in glass packages uses, e.g. during stacked storage or during closure application. Applied pressures can achieve 7 MPa in the last situation, generating tensile stresses on the shoulder and on the bottom. It has to be noted that glass bottles contain very often carbonated beverages, leading to differential pressure stresses across container walls (0.5–1.0 MPa). The weight and thickness of the final object can increase the resistance to such stresses with more efficacy than glass composition (Hambley 1986); heavy glass bottles, like those for sparkling wines, can resist internal pressure up to 7 MPa.

2.1.1.3   Optical Properties of Glass Packages

Glass packages are well known and appreciated for their transparency in the visible wavelengths range and to microwaves, leading to low energy dissipation, i.e. to negligible reduction in transmitted energy. Moreover, glass objects show very low ultraviolet (UV) transmission coefficients: this feature, often considered marginal, is more useful when speaking of quality protection of foods and beverages. These good properties are due both to the chemical nature of the ingredients and the acquired amorphous structure. The glass clearness may be modified by selecting appropriate metal oxides as minor ingredients, as well as the colour. Concerning UV transmission, the presence of alkaline oxides improves UV barriers provided by pure silica which, by itself, has a cut-off value around 150 nm.

2.1.2   Ceramics and Earthenware

Various materials, obtained by cooking a mixture of clay and water, are traditionally used to contain foods and beverages; they are variously indicated (not always properly) as ceramics, china, porcelain, pottery, stoneware, earthenware (Table 2.4). Clays are fine-grained soil, combined with hydrous aluminum phyllosilicates or other silicate minerals, traces of metal oxides and organic matter. Silicate minerals, the largest component, are easily available materials: they constitute approximately 90 % of the Earth's crust. These minerals are classified on the basis of their silicate structure, which may contain different ratios of silicon and oxygen.

Earthenware jars have been extensively used as food and beverage containers in ancient times by Greeks and Romans (Twede 2002). However, ceramic materials are still widely used for tableware, cookware and storage vessels. Several different types of these materials can be produced by selecting appropriate clays, water mixtures and the firing process.

Table 2.4 Tentative definitions of ceramics

Ceramic	Any article made of natural clay, non-metallic minerals mixed in various formulas with water and sometimes organic materials, shaped, processed or consolidated at high temperatures. Ceramic materials in contact with foods are used in all forms of pottery from crude earthenware to the finest porcelain
Pottery	It usually falls into three main classes: porous-bodied pottery, stoneware and porcelain. Raw clay is transformed into a porous pottery when it is heated at about 500 °C. Pottery commonly describes functional clay objects that serve a purpose in daily life (as plates, cups or vases)
Terracotta	Terracotta ('baked dirt' from the Latin *terra cotta*) is a type of red earthenware usually unglazed. The typical firing temperature is around 1000 °C. The iron content gives the fired body a brownish colour, which varies considerably being yellow, orange, red, *terracotta*, pink, grey or brown
Earthenware	It is made from either red or white clay baked at low temperature, typically 1,000–1,080 °C. Since it has not been fired to the point of vitrification, earthenware is porous and must be glazed in order to be watertight. It is generally more fragile than other types of pottery
Stoneware	Stoneware is composed of fire clay and ball clay as well as feldspar and silica. It is fired at high temperatures, typically 1,148–1,316 °C (2,100–2,400 °F), and is inherently non-porous. The white, grey or brown clay vitrifies during firing; so, the surface will be watertight. Stoneware is harder, stronger and more durable than earthenware
Porcelain	Porcelain is a white clay body used in making functional and non-functional pieces. Basically, the chemical composition of porcelain is a combination of clay, kaolin (a primary clay known for its translucency), feldspar, silica and quartz, but other materials may be added
Fine China	The fine china is fired at a lower temperature—around 1,200 °C (2,200 °F). Fine china is much softer than porcelain, making it much more suitable for applications such as plates and cups
Bone china	Bone china is a type of soft-paste porcelain made white and translucent by the addition of calcined animal bone to the body. The quality of the finished product is based on how much bone is in the mixture: a high-quality bone china should contain 30 to 40–45 % bone. Bone gives the fired body high levels of translucency and a unique milky white colour

Reproduced under permission from Bertolissi (2014)

A sharp classification is made into porous earthenware and non-porous porcelain (Chandler 1967; Hlavac 1983). Porous earthenware can be glazed for giving impermeability and brilliance obtaining china, porcelain and others products. A common way of manufacturing these containers involves drying of the wet shaped body, cooking at 800–1,000 °C. Finally, the manufacture is completed after a glazing or enamel coating through a 12 h—treatment at higher temperature (1,300–1,500 °C). Potteries of different glazing treatments are believed to play a fundamental role for attaining natural ripening in traditional oriental fermented foods.

Microporous earthenware are even more interesting because they may be tailored with controlled glazing or heating treatments to offer unique gas and moisture permeation properties (Seo et al. 2005). Carbon dioxide/oxygen permeability ratios close to unit may offer a new potential for respiring products packaging when these values are close to 1 (Kader et al. 1989). In addition, fermentation processes may be easily controlled (Yun et al. 2006). Furthermore, included metals have been supposed to act as low far—infrared emitters, leading to the inhibition of microbial growth (Vatansever and Hamblin 2012).

References

ASTM (2010) ASTM C162—05—Standard terminology of glass and glass products, ASTM vol 15.02 Glass; Ceramic Whitewares. ASTM International, West Conshohocken. doi:10.1520/C0162-05R10
Bertolissi N (2014) Are you able to tell the difference between porcelain and ceramic, or between fine china and bone china? http://www.nicolettabertolissi.com/difference-between-porcelain-and-ceramic/. Accessed 09 June 2015
Chandler M (1967) Ceramics in the modern world. Doubleday, Garden City
Chiang YM, Birnie D III, Kingery WD (1997) Physical ceramics—principles for ceramic science and engineering. Wiley, New York
Demuth T, Jeanvoine Y, Hafner J, Ángyán JG (1999) Polymorphism in silica studied in the local density and generalized-gradient approximations. J Phys: Condens Matter 11(19):3833. doi:10.1088/0953-8984/11/19/306
Hambley D (1986) Glass container design. In: Bakker M (ed) The Wiley encyclopedia of packaging technology. Wiley, New York
Hlavac J (1983) The technology of glass and ceramics. Elsevier Scientific, Amsterdam
Kader AA, Zagory D, Kerbel EL, Wang CY (1989) Modified atmosphere packaging of fruits and vegetables. Crit Rev Food Sci Nutr 28(1):1–30. doi:10.1080/10408398909527490
Lehman R (2004) Overview of glass properties. Glass Engineering 150:312. Rutgers University, Department of Ceramics and Materials Engineering. http://www.ifsc.usp.br/~lavfis2/BancoApostilasImagens/ApEfFotoelastico/Photoelastic-PropertyOverHandout.pdf. Accessed 05 June 2015
Mark HF, Bikales N, Overberger CG, Menges G, Kroschwitz JI (eds) (1985) Encyclopedia of Polymer science and engineering, 2nd edn. Wiley, New York
Nixon D (2015) Physical Properties. In: Scientific glassblowing shop. University of Delaware, 011 Brown Laboratory, Department of Chemistry and Biochemistry, Newark. http://www.udel.edu/chem/GlassShop/PhysicalProperties.htm#Vycor. Accessed 05 June 2015
Rawson H (1980) Properties and applications of glass. Elsevier, Amsterdam
Seo G, Chung S, An D, Lee D (2005) Permeabilities of Korean earthenware containers and their potential for packaging fresh produce. Food Sci Biotechnol 14(1):82–88
Twede D (2002) The packaging technology and science of ancient transport amphoras. Packag Technol Sci 15(4):181–195. doi:10.1002/pts.597
Varshneya AK (1994) Fundamentals of inorganic glasses. Academic Press, San Diego
Vatansever F, Hamblin M (2012) Far infrared radiation (FIR): its biological effects and medical applications. Photonics Lasers Med 1(4):255–266. doi:10.1515/plm-2012-0034
Yun JH, An DS, Lee K-E, Jun BS, Lee DS (2006) Modified atmosphere packaging of fresh produce using microporous earthenware material. Packag Technol Sci 19(5):269–278. doi:10.1002/pts.730
Zhao B, Yang P, Basir OA, Mittal GS (2006) Ultrasound based glass fragments detection in glass containers filled with beverages using neural networks and short time Fourier transform. Food Res Int 39(6):686–695. doi:10.1016/j.foodres.2006.01.008

Chapter 3
Metal Packaging Materials

Abstract The majority of known elements are metals. With relation to food packaging, these elements are used in a very pure form (aluminum) and as metal alloys (steel, tin plate). Five fundamental characteristics of metals make them particularly feasible for packaging: compactness, high density, unrivalled toughness, malleability and high thermal conductivity. In addition, the easiness of a selective collection of the metallic waste (due to magnetic behaviour and high density values) and the opportunity of thermal recycling without any loss of the original performances should be noted. As a result, three main classes of metallic materials for food packaging applications are currently available on the market: aluminum, coated plates (tinplate, tin-free steel, polymer-coated and steels) and stainless steel plates. Each material has interesting features on the one hand and peculiar disadvantages on the other side, when speaking of food packaging applications and other topics such as simple logistic considerations (oxidation, etc.).

Keywords Aluminum · Chromium · Iron · Lacquer · Metal packaging · Steel · Tin · Tin-free steel · Tinplate

Abbreviations

Al	Aluminum
Al_2O_3	Aluminum oxide
BPA	Bisphenol A
C	Carbon
Cr_2O_3	Chromic oxide
Cr	Chromium
ECCS	Electrolytically chromium-coated steel
EHEDG	European Hygiene Engineering and Design Group
FEP	Fluorinated perfluoroethylenepropylene
Fe	Iron
Fe/Sn	Iron/Tin
PFA	Perfluoroalkoxy alkane
PTFE	Polytetrafluoroethylene
Sn	Tin

© The Author(s) 2016
L. Piergiovanni and S. Limbo, *Food Packaging Materials*,
Chemistry of Foods, DOI 10.1007/978-3-319-24732-8_3

TFS   Tin-free steel
SnOx   Tin oxide

3.1 Metal Packaging Materials: An Overview

The majority (about three quarters) of known elements are metals. However, they are rarely found in a pure form; on the contrary, metals are combined mainly with oxygen, sulphur and silicon, to form ores. With relation to food packaging, these elements are used in a very pure form (aluminum) and as metal alloys (steel, tin plate). Therefore, the production of food packaging products starts from ores which are mined, then refined to extract the metal; its initial concentration in the mineral, as well as its form of occurrence, will directly affect costs associated with the final material. Five fundamental characteristics of metals make them particularly feasible for packaging.

First, the compactness of the molecular structure and the consequent high density can explain the impossibility of diffusive phenomena (light, vapour or gas) through very thin materials, leading to 'absolute barriers'. Second, the unrivalled toughness (that makes metal packages resistant against possible stress and abuse) has to be considered.

Moreover, the malleability, i.e. the possibility of moulding metals to reach almost any shape, is important: in other words, this property is the consequence of the metallic bonding among atoms. For the same reason, the high thermal conductivity—which makes feasible thermal treatments (pasteurisation, sterilisation) on the closed metal package to achieve the longest food shelf lives—should be discussed.

Finally, the easiness of a selective collection of the metallic waste (due to magnetic behaviour and high density values) and the opportunity of thermal recycling without any loss of the original performances should be noted.

Metal packaging products are, by far, cans and similar containers, but also closures, kegs, collapsible tubes and aerosol containers. In addition, thin flexible foils are produced when speaking of aluminum only. Since they can get in contact with a wide variety of different foods and beverages, a better comprehension of metals behaviour as packaging materials is opportune, particularly in critical applications (Parkar and Rakesh 2014).

Sometimes, minor metals occur in metal packaging construction (nickel, copper, titanium). However, main metallic materials (aluminum, tinplate, tin-free steel and stainless steel) only will be discussed in this section.

3.2 Aluminum

Aluminum is the third element in the Earth's crust (8.1 %) after oxygen and silicon. The main aluminum-containing mineral is bauxite, but many others contain aluminum oxide, together with oxides of silicon, iron and other metals. The production of pure aluminum is an electrolytic process applied to aluminum oxide (Al_2O_3) obtained from ores.

Aluminum production is not cheap: consequently, this metal is the most expensive material used for food packaging purposes. One kg of aluminum takes about 4 kg of mineral and requires seven to tenfold the energy needed by the same mass of iron. The reason is that aluminum reactions with oxygen and other elements are thermodynamically favourite, while counter reactions are not at all. As a result, the reduction of aluminum to pure metal requires a huge amount of energy.

On the other hand, because of the spontaneous reaction of this metal with oxygen, the formation of a thin passivated film (1–5 nm) can be obtained. This result can be very useful because of the slight protection to the corrosion phenomena. Since the oxidised layer is thin and not uniform, aluminum sheets are preferably processed by a chemical or electrochemical passivation (anodisation) which increases the thickness to 50–200 nm. This spontaneous or chemical passivation of the metal, that protects the metal from corrosion, is removable both at low (<4.0) and at high (>8.0) pH values (Davis 1999); more details on metal corrosion are provided in Sect. 7.2. With concern to the necessity of improving the corrosion resistance of final aluminum packages, as food packaging is concerned, the metal surface is often protected by lacquers or polymer coatings.

Several different aluminum alloys are used for packaging production, but they are always very rich in aluminum concentration. In particular, two elements are considered when differentiating these alloys: manganese and magnesium.

Magnesium increases the mechanical resistance of materials but reduces corrosion resistance against acids and alkalis. Manganese slightly increases the corrosion resistance. Table 3.1 shows the main types of aluminum alloys with main compositions and specific uses which are related to physical properties of the final material.

Table 3.1 Main aluminum alloys and composition (%) as function of the final use (Alcoa 2006; Lee et al. 2008; Morris 2011; Sanders et al. 1989)

Alloy code	Use	Mn	Si	Fe	Mg	Cu	Cr
1050	Foils and flexible tubes	0.05	0.25	0.4	–	0.05	–
3004	Body stock	1.00–1.50	0.18–0.30	0.4–0.7	0.80–1.3	0.25	–
5182	End stock	0.20–0.50	0.20	0.35	4.0 0–5.00	0.06	0.10
5052		0.10	0.45	0.45	2.20–2.80	0.10	0.15–0.35
5042	Tab stock	0.20–0.50	0.20	0.35	3.00–4.00	0.15	0.10
5082		0.15	0.20	0.35	4.00–5.00	0.15	0.15
8079	Foils for lamination	–			–	0.05	–

3.2.1 Mechanical Properties of Aluminum Packaging Materials

Two physical properties of aluminum (Al) are well known: Al is the lightest metal (density around 2.7 g cm^{-3}) and has an extraordinary malleability (according to the alloy components) that makes it possible to reduce the thickness of aluminum foils even to 3.0 μm. These properties allow to cast Al in any forms, to roll it, and extrude it into a variety of shapes making easy the manufacturing of aluminum packaging.

Above mentioned effects of magnesium and manganese permit to prepare alloys with very different mechanical properties. These materials can:

- Act as thin wrappings (for chocolates)
- Be deeply drowned (when speaking of 'two-pieces' cans)
- Reach the high rigidity required by easy opening devices.

Anyway, all aluminum alloys used in packaging have Al contents ≥95 %. For this reason, recycling processes are easy and convenient: the production of aluminum packages, using recycled metals, uses only 5 % of the energy used in primary production.

3.2.2 Thermal Properties of Aluminum Packaging Materials

All the thermal properties of Al result very useful for food packaging applications. At temperatures below zero, aluminum strength increases and even at ultra-freezing temperatures it does not become fragile; consequently, aluminum is an extremely useful low-temperature material. Moreover, its thermal conductivity is very high and higher than all the other metals used in packaging (Table 3.2); therefore, a pasteurisation or sterilisation treatment applied on an Al package will be more effective and less energy consuming.

Table 3.2 Thermal properties of some metal packaging materials (Lee et al. 2008; Mondolfo 1976)

Property	Aluminum	Carbon steel	Stainless steel (austenitic type)
Mass thermal capacity (kJ kg^{-1} °C^{-1})	0.90	0.45–2.08	0.420–0.500
Thermal expansion α (°C^{-1} × °C 10^{-6})	24	11–16.6	9.0–20.7
Thermal conductivity (W m^{-1} °C^{-1} at 25 °C)	237	24.3–65.2	11.2–36.7
Melting temperature (°C)	600–670	1426–1538	1371–1454
Boiling temperature (°C)	2476.8–2518.8	–	–

The melting temperature of whatever aluminum alloy is lower than 700 °C. In addition, the possibility of evaporating pure aluminum (about 1,500 °C) at very low pressures (1.333–0.0133 Pa) is extremely important. Thus, it is possible to obtain the condensation of aluminum onto various flexible substrates (plastic films, paper sheets) as a very thin layer of some tenths or hundreds of nm. As a result, metallised flexible materials can be produced for interesting applications in packaging because of their low transparency and low permeability to gas and vapour (Piergiovanni and Limbo 2004).

3.3 Coated Steels

Many iron (Fe) alloys are named 'steels'. They represent the most used structural metallic materials in constructions and in the packaging sector too, in detail, they are the most common material for metal packaging productions. All of them have a carbon (C) content ranging from 0.2 to 2 %: carbon has a fundamental binding role in the alloy, securing the atoms of iron in a quite rigid lattice and, thus, establishing final properties of the steel. In particular, both the tensile strength and the brittleness of the final material are enhanced increasing the carbon content.

Iron alloys may be different for crystallographic structures and for the content of various metal elements—manganese, chromium, nickel, molybdenum, copper, tungsten, cobalt and silicon—leading to a great number of different compositions and performance. The most common alloys in the food packaging sector belong to the family of so-called 'carbon steels': generally, they contain manganese (e.g. 1.6 %), silicon (e.g. 0.6 %), copper (e.g. 0.6 %), phosphorous (e.g. 0.4 %), sulphur (e.g. 0.05 %) and C does not exceed 1 %. Thermal properties of carbon steels are shown in Table 3.2 while Table 3.3 compares the average mechanical properties of a carbon steel to other metallic packaging materials.

Steels are known as cheap, strong, hard, durable and easy to shape materials; however, they are not enough inert for food contact applications. In fact, coated steels only are used in food packaging productions.

Table 3.3 Mechanical properties of some metal packaging materials (Lee et al. 2008; Veschi 1989)

Property	Aluminum	Carbon steel	Stainless steel (austenitic type)
Mass per unit volume (g cm^{-3})	2.64–3.20	7.85	7.75–8.1
Static coefficient of friction	1.9	–	–
Modulus of elasticity (GPa)	67.5–70	190–210	190–210
Tensile strength (MPa)	70–210	276–1882	640–2000

3.3.1   Tinplate

By far, the most important coated steel in food packaging applications is tinplate. Along a thickness ranging approximately between 0.13 and 0.40 mm, tinplate presents the structure depicted in Fig. 3.1, which is the consequence of physical (thermal and mechanical) and chemical (electrolytic coating, oxidation, lubrication) steps of preparation (Morgan and Hopkins 1985). The most important steps for the required inertness are tin coating (tinning) and passivation properties. The 'tinning' is made by an electrolytic process where the steel is covered by a thin layer of metallic tin (Sn) in a bath of tin sulphate in sulphuric acid. This step is followed by a thermal treatment (260–270 °C) and a rapid quenching that leads to the formation of the iron/tin (Fe/Sn) alloy. The subsequent step is the chemical passivation that takes place in a solution of sodium dichromate where tin and chromium oxides and tin oxides (SnOx) are produced on surfaces. Finally, an oily lubricant (e.g. acetyl tributyl citrate or dioctyl sebacate) is applied to enhance the protection against surface scratch and the resistance to environmental corrosion.

The tinplate has a good but not total inertness (see also Sect. 7.2); therefore, the material is very often further protected with organic coatings, inside and outside the body and ends of the final container (Barilli et al. 2003). The grammage of these coating ranges from 3 to 9 g m^{-2}, leading to thicknesses that range from 4 to 12 μm.

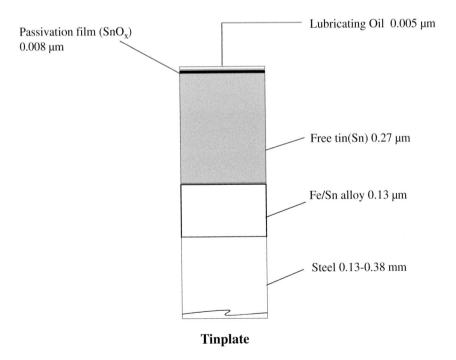

Passivation film (SnO$_x$) 0.008 μm

Lubricating Oil 0.005 μm

Free tin(Sn) 0.27 μm

Fe/Sn alloy 0.13 μm

Steel 0.13-0.38 mm

Tinplate

Fig. 3.1 The section structure of tinplate after physical and chemical manufacturing steps

These coatings are called lacquers or enamels: they are chemically quite different. Moreover, their properties are extremely important during the can manufacturing (e.g. for the deep drawing required to obtain 'two pieces' cans) and with relation to possible food packaging interactions. Most common lacquers are:

- Oleoresinous coatings of natural origin, blended with various components including zinc oxide for sulphur-containing foods, such as corn and meat products
- Vinyl-type lacquers, made by dissolving vinyl chloride and vinyl acetate copolymer in solvents. They do not have any taste and odour, are resistant against acid, alkali, oil and detergent but not very heat stable. Therefore, these products are used for canned dry foods, beers, and beverages. On the other hand, they are not recommended when speaking of retorted foods
- Phenolic lacquers. These products are resistant to oil, acid, and sulphide staining; they are often used in combination as epoxy-phenolic coatings
- Epoxy resins, produced from condensation polymerisation between epichlorohydrin and bisphenol A. They are one of the most widely used coatings in metal cans, in particular for acidic and non-acid foods and beverages (fruits, vegetables, meats, fishes, juices, beers, and soft drinks). Recently, there has been a rise in attention about the risk of migration of bisphenol A (BPA) from epoxy-type coating. BPA is suspected to be an endocrine disruptor (Shelnutt et al. 2013; Cunha and Fernandes 2013)
- Acrylics coatings (derived from the polymerisation of acrylic acid and its derivatives. These products provide good colour retention and heat stability. They are often applied as epoxy-acrylates in water-based spray coatings
- Polyester coatings (also named 'alkyd' resins) are produced by esterification between an alcohol, such as glycerol or penta-erythritol, and a polybasic acid or anhydride, such as phthalic anhydride. These lacquers are used more for external coating than for internal lacquering.

3.3.2 Tin-Free Steel

Because of limited availability and high costs, the development of 'Tin-Free Steel' (TFS), i.e. plates protected with a layer of different metal oxide, took place since 1960s. The best alternative to tinplate is the electrolytically chromium-coated steel (ECCS): this product is obtained with chromium and chromium oxide. In fact, chromium is one of the few metals that have the property of spontaneous passivation (see also Sect. 3.4). The passivation layer is thinner than the multilayered structure of $SnOx$; in addition, it is compact and hard. As a consequence, the ECCS plate has even better functionality in heat resistance, coating adhesion and printing. ECCS is less resistant than tinplate to corrosion in acidic environment, but more resistant at neutral or alkaline pH values. However, the use of ECCS in food packaging is much more limited than tinplate: this material is mainly recommended for food can ends, crown caps, vacuum closures for glass preserve jars (International Icon Group 2009).

3.3.3 Polymer-Coated Steels

The most recent evolution of coated steels for packaging applications is correlated to polymer-coated plates. Synthetic thermo-plastic polymers can be successfully applied directly on steel plates, as well as on already coated tinplate or ECCS for further protection against corrosion. Different polymers—e.g. polytetrafluoroethylene (PTFE), perfluoroalkoxy alkane (PFA), fluorinated perfluoroethylenepropylene (FEP)—with various thicknesses can be simultaneously coated or laminated onto opposite surfaces (Leivo et al. 2004). In addition to the excellent appearance, advantages of polymer-coated steels are resistance against abrasion, corrosion and food interactions, as well as outstanding moisture barrier (Boelen et al. 2004; Ohtsuka 2012).

3.4 Stainless Steels

The corrosion resistance of these kinds of iron alloys, named 'stainless steels', is so high that they can get in contact with any food and beverage (but also many chemicals) without any further protection or covering. The outstanding chemical inertness is provided by the content of chromium (Cr) which is always higher than 11 %. While Cr is a moderately active metal, it reacts at room temperature with oxygen in air to form Cr (III); chromic oxide (Cr_2O_3) is also one of the most common form of Cr naturally occurring in minerals. This state of auto-passivation protects the alloy from corrosion, both at the surface and in the mass of the material. A great number of different stainless steel are known and internationally classified: they differ on the basis of their crystalline structure (austenitic, ferritic, and martensitic states) and according to their alloy composition. Austenitic types are the most common states in packaging applications; some of their main physical properties are reported in Tables 3.2 and 3.3. Because of their economic value, stainless steels are only used in food packaging as returnable containers for beverages (kegs for beers, wines, cokes, …). On the other side, they are the leading materials for large storage industrial-containers, as well as for processing plants, kitchen tools, and many other objects intended for food contact.

Table 3.4 lists some typical applications of various stainless steel materials in the food industry. Even if the most recognised characteristic of stainless steels is the chemical inertness, many other properties deserve to be mentioned. These steels have high resilience, good thermal conductivity, ease of welding, and outstanding hygienic properties. Research works conducted on artificially contaminated

Table 3.4 Typical applications of the various stainless steel materials in the food industry (Cvetkovski 2012; EHEDG 2005; Newson 2001)

Types	Main uses
Austenitic 304 steel	A certain attitude to formability and weldability may be required. In addition, produced pieces—bowls, machinery components, etc.—should have corrosion resistance performances superior to 430 ferritic steels
Austenitic 316 steel	A notable corrosion resistance is required: components are used with moderately corrosive foods (meat/blood, products with a certain salt content). In addition, obtained pieces have to be frequently washed/cleaned. On the other side, stationary solids and excessive stress are not expected
Austenitic 1,4539 steel	A notable corrosion resistance is required: components are used with highly corrosive foods (stagnant salty foods, etc.)
Duplex 1,4462 steel	Excellent corrosion resistance is required in comparison with austenitics: components are used with highly corrosive foods (stagnant salty foods, etc.). In addition, these duplex steels (1.4462 and 1.4362 also) are used when good resistance values to stress corrosion cracking in salt solutions is needed at high temperatures
Austenitic 6 % Mo-types	Excellent corrosion resistance is required in comparison with austenitics: components are used with highly corrosive foods (stagnant salty foods, etc.). In addition, these duplex steels (1.4462 and 1.4362 also) are used when good resistance values to stress corrosion cracking in salt solutions is needed at high temperatures. These superaustenitic are recommended for permanent immersion in seawater (hot water boilers, etc.)
420 Martensitic steel	Professional knives, spatulas similar cooking instruments, etc.
430 Ferritic steel	Production of instruments and components for moderately corrosive environments (e.g. vegetables, drinks, etc.). Several examples are table surfaces, equipment cladding and other products. Little formability or weldability is required when speaking of these products

materials have clearly demonstrated the higher bacterial removing capacity of standard cleaning processes on stainless steel. They show a low bacterial retention, probably related to the difficulty of biofilm formation onto its glossy surface (Arnold and Bailey 2000).

References

Alcoa (2006) Global product specifications. Alcoa Inc., Rigid Container Sheet. https://www.alcoa.com/mill_products/catalog/pdf/China_Specs/Can_Sheet_Specs.pdf. Accessed 09 June 2015

Arnold JW, Bailey GW (2000) Surface finishes on stainless steel reduce bacterial attachment and early biofilm formation: scanning electron and atomic force microscopy study. Poult Sci 79 (12):1839–1845. doi:10.1093/ps/79.12.1839

Barilli F, Fragni R, Gelati S, Montanari A (2003) Study on the adhesion of different types of lacquers used in food packaging. Prog Org Coat 46(2):91–96. doi:10.1016/S0300-9440(02)00215-1

Boelen B, den Hartog H, van der Weijde H (2004) Product performance of polymer coated packaging steel, study of the mechanism of defect growth in cans. Prog Org Coat 50(1):40–46. doi:10.1016/j.porgcoat.2003.09.011

Cvetkovski C (2012) Stainless steel in contact with food and beverage. Metall Mater Eng 18 (4):283–293

Cunha SC, Fernandes JO (2013) Assessment of bisphenol A and bisphenol B in canned vegetables and fruits by gas chromatography–mass spectrometry after QuEChERS and dispersive liquid–liquid microextraction. Food Control 33(2):549–555. doi:10.1016/j.foodcont.2013.03.028

Davis JR (1999) Corrosion of aluminum and aluminum alloys. ASM International, Materials Park

EHEDG (2005) Materials of construction for equipment in contact with food. European Hygiene Engineering and Design Group, Frankfurt/Main

International Icon Group (2009) The 2009 report on tin-free steel carbon steel tin mill products: World Market ICON Group International, Inc. Las Vegas, USA

Lee DS, Yam KL, Piergiovanni L (2008) Metal packaging. In: Lee DS, Yam KL, Piergiovanni L (eds) Food packaging science and technology. CRC Press, Boca Raton

Leivo E, Wilenius T, Kinos T, Vuoristo P, Mäntylä T (2004) Properties of thermally sprayed fluoropolymer PVDF, ECTFE, PFA and FEP coatings. Progr Org Coat 49(1):69–73. doi:10.1016/j.porgcoat.2003.08.011

Mondolfo LF (1976) Aluminum alloys structure and properties, p 56. Butterworth & Co., London

Morgan E, Hopkins DW (1985) Tinplate and modern canmaking technology. The pergamon materials engineering practice series. Elsevier, London

Morris SA (2011) Food and package engineering. Wiley, New York

Newson T (2001) Stainless steel-applications, grades and human exposure. AvestaPolarit Oyj Abp, Espoo

Ohtsuka T (2012) Corrosion protection of steels by conducting polymer coating. Int J Corros 2012:1–7. doi:10.1155/2012/915090

Parkar J, Rakesh M (2014) Leaching of elements from packaging material into canned foods marketed in India. Food Control 40:177–184. doi:10.1016/j.foodcont.2013.11.042

Piergiovanni L, Limbo S (2004) The protective effect of film metallization against oxidative deterioration and discoloration of sensitive foods. Packag Technol Sci 17(3):155–164. doi:10.1002/pts.651

Sanders RE, Baumann SF Jr, Stumpf HC (1989) Wrought non-heat-treatable aluminum alloys. In: Vasudevan AK, Doherty RD (eds) Aluminum alloys—contemporary research and applications. Academic Press, San Diego

Shelnutt S, Kind J, Allaben W (2013) Bisphenol A: update on newly developed data and how they address NTP's 2008 finding of 'Some Concern'. Food Chem Toxicol 57:284–295. doi:10.1016/j.fct.2013.03.027

Veschi D (1989) L'Alluminio e le leghe leggere, p 8. Ulrico Hoepli Editore, Milan

Chapter 4
Cellulosic Packaging Materials

Abstract The most abundant biopolymers in the biosphere are carbohydrates polymers which account for three-fourth of the global available biomass. Cellulose is, by far, the most abundant and widely spread carbohydrates polymer and the first renewable organic material. The packaging industry uses cellulose-based materials on a very large scale: these matters represent the biggest part of the whole packaging materials in all countries. Actually, cellulosic packaging is quite a broad category of different types including both primary and secondary packages, as well as wrapping materials and containers. In fact, even if the basic chemical structure of cellulose is the same in all the different cellulosic materials, their final structure can be significantly dissimilar. This variability, due to a combination of cellulose biosynthesis conditions and technological features, allows to obtain different packaging products: papers, boards, regenerated cellulose (cellophane), moulded cellulose, etc. General features of main cellulosic packaging materials are strictly linked with cellulose chemistry.

Keywords Biopolymer · Carbohydrate · Cellulose · Corrugated board · Hemicellulose · Lignin · Nanocellulose · Paperboard · Regenerated cellulose

Abbreviations

CNCs	Cellulose nanocrystals
DP	Degree of polymerisation
OH	Hydroxyl
MW	Molecular weight
MFC	Microfibrillated cellulose
NFC	Nanofibrillated cellulose

4.1 Cellulosic Packaging Materials. An Overview

The most abundant biopolymers in the biosphere are carbohydrates polymers which account for 75 % of the global available biomass. Cellulose is, by far, the most abundant and widely spread carbohydrates polymer and the first renewable organic

© The Author(s) 2016
L. Piergiovanni and S. Limbo, *Food Packaging Materials*,
Chemistry of Foods, DOI 10.1007/978-3-319-24732-8_4

material, accounting yearly for more than 75 billion tonnes (French et al. 2004). The packaging industry uses cellulose-based materials on a very large scale: these matters represent the biggest part (around 40 %) of the whole packaging materials in all countries (Piergiovanni 2009).

Actually, cellulosic packaging is quite a broad category of different types including both primary and secondary packages, as well as wrapping materials and containers (Lee et al. 2008). This large assortment of different uses and properties comes from various factors including chemical additives used in their manufacturing: cellulosic packaging materials are always heterogeneous solids, where the cellulose content can be even lower than 50 % by weight. Further, in order to understand the features and potential uses in packaging of various cellulosic materials, it is also relevant to realise the importance of the supramolecular organisation of cellulose, deriving from different sources and processes. In fact, even if the basic chemical structure of cellulose is the same in all the different cellulosic materials, their final structure can be significantly dissimilar. This variability is due to a combination of cellulose biosynthesis conditions, as well as chemical and physical consequences of technologies used for arranging them in a network matrix, i.e. the three-dimensional cellulose fibres complex, set in papers, boards, regenerated cellulose (cellophane) or moulded cellulose. In this section, the general characteristics of main cellulosic packaging materials will be described after a short discussion of cellulose chemistry and its reduction to nanodimensions, which is one of the most promising trends in this sector.

4.1.1 Basic Cellulose Chemistry and Morphology

Since 1926, it is known that cellulose is a high-molecular-weight, linear homopolymer of β-1,4-linked anhydro-D-glucose (Staudinger 1926). Glucose residues are inverted 180° in the linear polymer, leading to a fundamental dimer unit, named 'cellobiose' and shown in Fig. 4.1. Molecular weights (MW) of cellulose polymer are in the range of 540–2,700 kDa, due to chain lengths in the range of 3,000–15,000 anhydro-glucoses units. Extensive hydrogen bonds can be formed between the parallel chains, resulting in the formation of insoluble microfibrils, which are in turn assembled into cellulose fibres. According to the source material, the dimension of fibres may be very different, ranging from 0.7 to 4.5 mm in width and 20–45 mm in length when speaking of woods. Dislocations are always possible along cellulose chains in the microfibrils, leading to regions of different symmetry: the substantially disordered regions are called the amorphous part. The crystalline parts are the ones relatively high in crystallinity, with only a low number (5–30 %) of dislocated chains and with strongly packed chains.

The possible chemical reactions of cellulose are mostly those related to the cleavage of the β-1,4 glycosidic bond and to the possible reactivity of hydroxyl (OH) groups. The acidic hydrolysis of glycosidic linkages is much more effective on the amorphous parts of native cellulose which are less dense. The hydrolysing attack

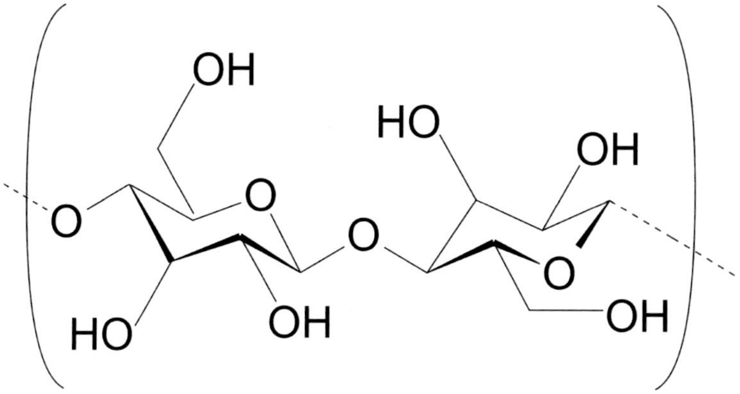

Fig. 4.1 The linear monomer of β-1,4- linked anhydro-D-glucose in the cellulose structure (cellobiose). BKchem version 0.13.0, 2009 (http://bkchem.zirael.org/index.html) has been used for drawing this structure

leaves crystalline particles with shorter chains and it is a good way to reach nanodimensions and to produce cellulosic nanoparticles that will be discussed later. During an acid hydrolysis processes, the degree of polymerisation (DP) of cellulose quickly reduces until a quite constant value around a range of 100–300 DP, because of the almost null sensitivity of crystalline regions to acid attacks. However, the glycosidic cleavage is also possible by means of enzymatic processes, using e.g. commercially available cellulases and endoglucanases (Meyabadi and Dadashian 2012).

The reactivity of OH– groups can be very useful to change the surface chemistry, introducing different chemical moieties by esterification, oxidation and other possible reactions. Actually, only –CH_2–OH– groups (Fig. 4.1) and partially the one OH– group in position 2 of anhydro-glucoses units are available for reacting because of the $^4C_1$ chair conformation adopted by cellulose (Roy et al. 2009). Acetylation is, by far, the most classic and common way of changing cellulose chemistry. Cellulose acetate has been used in photography, as a synthetic fibre, as packaging material and in many other applications.

Besides the chemical changes of cellulose, related to possible covalent bonding on the –OH moiety, the electrostatic interactions should be also mentioned. Transformations led through adsorption phenomena onto the cellulose polymer exhibit interesting performance with respect to packaging materials. The charge density of native cellulose is quite low; however, polyelectrolytes have long been used as dry and wet strength or antistatic additives in paper manufacturing, including other pertinent uses with relation to the packaging sector. Both the chemical changes and the electrostatic interactions are also promising ways to enhance the opportunity of useful applications of nanocellulose. The introduction of cellulose in the 'nano' form has very interesting potential applications in various industrial sectors and particularly in packaging, allowing the development of novel materials, as well as the improvement of conventional materials performances. Together with fundamental aspects such as its renewable nature, biodegradability and nonfood

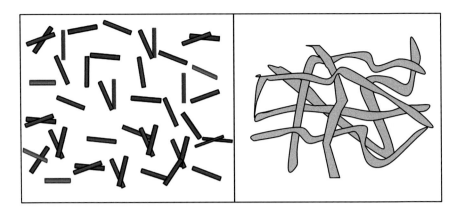

Cellulose nanocrystals (CNCs)   Nanofibrillated Cellulose (NFC)

Fig. 4.2 Cellulose nanoparticles obtained by different processes: acidic hydrolysis (CNCs) and mechanical treatments (NFC)

agricultural-based sources, the use of nanocellulose has recently attracted a huge attention in the field of packaging materials (Li et al. 2015). A nano-sized phase, alone or included in a different matrix, will result in a great increase of interfaces, enhancing mechanical and barrier properties of final materials.

Nanocellulose can be used as filler in composites manufacture, as a coating of conventional films and papers and as self-standing thin films. As above mentioned, the acidic hydrolysis is the preferable route in order to obtain cellulose nanocrystals (CNCs); besides this method, mechanical processes are also already in use to reach nanodimensions and to obtain nanoparticles of cellulose. Mechanical treatments require more energy with respect to the acid hydrolysis process, leading to a bigger amount of amorphous particles with higher aspect ratio, in an extensively entangled network. In these processes, high shear stresses are provided by different means (mainly by various steps of high-pressure homogeniser) in order to induce transverse cleavage along the cellulose microfibrillar structure. Obtained products are long and thin cellulose fibrils, termed microfibrillated cellulose (MFC) or nanofibrillated cellulose (NFC), according to final dimensions (Fig. 4.2); these dimensions, for NFC and CNCs, are generally in the range of 5–25 nm in width and 50–250 nm in length.

4.2   Papers and Boards

From a general viewpoint, papers and solid boards are manufactured from the same starting materials and by the same papermaking process, at least in the preliminary steps (Kirwan 2011). The main constituents of major cellulosic packaging materials come from wood fibres: cellulose, hemicellulose and lignin. For their importance, lignin and hemicellulose also deserve to be shortly described after cellulose.

4.2.1 Lignin

Within the fibre structure of all lignocellulosic sources (and exclusively in them), lignin forms a cementing matrix that holds together cellulose fibrils and give them an outstanding mechanical resistance. Lignin is a highly branched, amorphous polymer with a very high degree of polymerisation of alkyl aromatic molecules; the structure of these compounds is different in various plant species (chemical reasons are not completely cleared). The complete removal of lignin among fibrils is not always easy in the papermaking process: this is a serious problem because, reacting with used chemicals, lignin leads to dark brown soluble derivatives. Therefore, bleaching processes are quite often necessary to increase the whiteness of the final materials.

The oxidation of coloured substances, a needed step when speaking of enhanced brightness, is obtained by chlorinated chemicals (chlorine, hypochlorite and chlorine dioxide) and oxygenated substances (oxygen, ozone, hydrogen peroxide). Bleaching processes, which are often questioned for their possible pollution, may also reduce tensile properties of final materials.

4.2.2 Hemicellulose

Hemicellulose consists of amorphous copolymers of one or more sugars such as xylose, mannose, arabinose and galactose, combined with uronic acids. Due to an average low MW and low DP (100–200), hemicelluloses are highly soluble in diluted alkali and, therefore, easily separated from cellulose in the pulping process. However, a higher content of hemicellulose increases greatly tensile, burst and folding strengths of the final materials; moisture uptake is greater in cellulosic materials with higher hemicelluloses.

4.2.3 The Pulping Process

The pulping process is the operation to transform raw materials (usually wood chips) into an intermediate (pulp) rich in cellulose fibres. At present, different technologies for pulping are in use according to the fibres source and desired features of the final packaging material.

The cheapest technology with the highest yield is the so-called mechanical pulping. This process does not require any chemicals but a fast rotating grindstone against which wooden chips are forced, while the heat generated is removed by a continuous casting of water. Obtained pulp contains a large quantity of lignin and many other wood constituents. Frequently, also some refining steps are included in this mechanical pulping process which is used in the manufacture of some strong papers and papers for corrugated board construction.

The most common chemical processes consist of cellulose refining steps resulting in lower yield and better quality. The most important process is the sulphate method, also known as 'kraft' (this word means 'strong' in Swedish language) because of high mechanical properties of produced papers. The process uses solutions of sodium hydroxide, sulphite and sulphate. However, obtained cellulosic materials are brown in colour and additional bleaching processes are needed.

The sulphite process, instead, provides whiter products and higher yields. In this process, a solution of sodium sulphite and sulphurous acid is used, at pH values ranging between 1.5 and 5.0. Both the sulphate and the sulphite processes are able to dissolve lignin, but the first is much more effective in an alkaline environment. Chemical, thermal and mechanical processes can be also combined to achieve the goal of a complete liberation of cellulose fibres from crusted substances of plant sources. The rationale is to combine and optimise the peculiarities of each one in saving the fibre integrity, accelerating the process and controlling costs and yields of the final product.

4.2.4 Papermaking

The diluted pulp (5–7 % of solid content) is always submitted to a mechanical operation, called beating or refining, with the aim of increasing the interfibres bonding, mainly by a low water absorption. The future physical properties of paper bags or folding cartons are largely influenced by this operation. Hemicelluloses in the pulp have a great importance in this step as they are located close to cellulose chains and they swell quickly, leading to fibres that are more flexible and more suitable for subsequent papermaking operations.

Furthermore, the beating/refining step is also the one where non-fibrous additives are added. Several chemical substances are commonly used in the manufacturing of cellulosic packaging materials to increase performance (Table 4.1). Occasionally, some sensorial and potential safety problems of packaged foods are related to the transfer of such chemicals, particularly in recycled papers and boards (Guazzotti et al. 2014, 2015).

Once the refining process is completed, the chemical composition of cellulosic materials is established on a dry base, but still in a diluted water suspension. The further step is to cast the suspension onto the machine where the consolidation of cellulosic sheets occurs by draining it onto a fine flat screen or on rotating wire mesh cylinder connected to vacuum pumps.

The thickness of produced sheets depends on the suspension concentration and determines its grammage ($g\ m^{-2}$), i.e. the mass of the unit surface, which is the main

Table 4.1 Non-fibrous additives used in the paper making process

Category	Additives
Filler	Calcium carbonate, silicates, talc, barium sulphate, kaolin, Celite, etc.
Sizing	Rosin, rosin soap, glues, synthetic resins, waxes, silicones, carboxymethyl cellulose, starch, etc.
Surface sizing	Modified starches, styrene maleic anhydride, styrene acrylic emulsion, styrene acrylic acid, ethylene acrylic acid, gelatin, polyurethane, etc.
Colouring	Titanium oxide, optical brighteners, acid, basic or direct dyes, calcium carbonate; solvent vehicles may be included
Wet and dry strength	Formaldehyde resins, epichlorohydrin, glyoxal, gums, polyamines, phenolics, polyacrylamides, polyamides, cellulose derivatives, etc.
Technological aids	Antifoaming, draining, floating, chelating agents, etc.
Coating, adhesives, plasticisers	Aluminum hydroxide, polyvinyl acetate, acrylics, linseed oil, gums, protein glues, wax emulsions, azite, glyoxal, stearates, solvents, polyethylene, cellulose derivatives, foil, rubber derivatives, polyamines, polyesters, butadiene–styrene polymers, etc.
Other additives	Softeners, strengtheners, flame retardant, antimicrobial agents, etc.

criteria used worldwide to discriminate between papers and paperboards. The used apparatus also permits to give various textures on one or both sides of the material; however, many more 'finishing' grades are obtained with subsequent 'sheet drying' steps. In fact, when sheets leave the machine (moisture content is around 75–90 %), they need to be submitted to drying steps which are both mechanical pressing and thermal treatments. The small water that remains in the final cellulosic materials, is both bonded to cellulose and free in the interstices of fibres; this reduced aqueous amount has a great importance for ultimate package properties.

The moisture content can affect the dimensional stability and the mechanical resistance, as well as the shelf life of sensitive products. After drying steps, surface properties and the appearance can be further changed by other operations. In fact, various specific functions of food packaging cellulosic materials (sealability, moisture, oil and gas resistance) are obtained by means of coating, impregnating, laminating and finishing processes that take place commonly in different specialised companies. According to these converting techniques, a great number of different cellulosic materials are currently available, whose description is beyond the scope of this book.

4.3   Cellophane and Minor Materials

Chemical additives and treatments can further and notably extend the panorama of packaging materials, based on cellulose fibres (Yam 2009). The word 'greaseproof' refers to papers that offer resistance to fat and oil penetration, useful for wrapping fatty foods. They can be obtained through a very prolonged beating, leading to an extensive fibres rupture and the closure of interstitial voids. Better performance can be achieved by resin saturation or by coating with synthetic materials.

'Glassine' is a glossy, almost transparent paper, fairly resistant to oil and slightly brittle. It is produced by a mechanical and thermal process of a greaseproof paper. Both compression and heat promote massive hydrogen bonds among the inter-fibre matrix giving the final specific properties. Glassine-type papers are widely used in food contact applications, for bakery and confectionery products.

'Vegetable parchments' have surprising performance when speaking of fat and water resistance without any specific additive: a chemical process is required. Papers produced from chemical pulp are rapidly immerged (10–15 s) in sulphuric acid (65 %) at low temperature (10–15 °C). This treatment leads the fibres to swell and partially to dissolve leading to a gel which fills and glues interfibre voids. After the acid cure, the paper is washed (in alkaline solution and fresh water) to eliminate any chemicals; subsequently, it is dried to obtain high wet strength and resistance to grease and oils.

'Cellophane', also named 'regenerated cellulose', was invented in 1908 by E. Brandenberger (a Swiss textile engineer) who developed a completely new material by a complex chemical transformation of a pure cellulose pulp. This material has been for many years, the only transparent wrapping product with packaging applications.

The manufacturing process foresees a sequential treatment with caustic soda solution and carbon disulphide of the pulp; consequently, fibres are partially dissolved with the partial depolymerisation of cellulose. Then the viscose obtained is casted in a sulphuric acid and sodium sulphate bath to obtain the regeneration of a linear polymer of cellulose in a solid form. After steps of purification, softening and drying, the intermediate becomes the well-known clear film of cellophane. The very interesting mechanical and oxygen barrier properties of cellophane depend on the viscosity of the slurry (the degree of depolymerisation) and the softening step. Uncoated cellophane has no applications in food packaging for its high moisture sensitivity. On the other side, coated cellophane materials have still many applications in food packaging despite a higher price in comparison with synthetic plastic films of similar performance. The most common coatings are polyvinylidene chloride and nitrocellulose which provide thermosealability and high moisture resistance.

Among the minor cellulosic packaging materials, 'moulded cellulose' deserves to be mentioned because it is the only non-plane but three-dimensional cellulose object currently available. In fact, corrugated boards, bags, sachets, pouches and boxes are obtained by folding and gluing sheets of paper, boards or laminates of cellulosic materials, but the network of cellulose fibres can also be moulded in three-dimensional packages. These packages are obtained by squeezing aqueous fibre suspensions onto screen moulds to remove water. Some natural or synthetic glues might be added in the manufacturing process. Their production, therefore, is quite cheap, also for the possible use of recycled matter. They can be easily recycled after use too. Nevertheless, these packages have also interesting functional properties for their shock absorption ability and high transpiration rates that may be especially useful for 'respiring' products such as fresh fruits and vegetables.

References

French A, Bertoniere N, Brown R, Chanzy H, Gray D, Hattori K, Glasser W (2004) Cellulose. In: Seidel A (ed) Kirk-Othmer encyclopedia of chemical technology, vol. 5, 5th edn. Wiley, New York

Guazzotti V, Limbo S, Piergiovanni L, Fengler R, Fiedler D, Gruber L (2015) A study into the potential barrier properties against mineral oils of starch-based coatings on paperboard for food packaging. Food Packag Shelf Life 3:9–18. doi:10.1016/j.fpsl.2014.09.003

Guazzotti V, Marti A, Piergiovanni L, Limbo S (2014) Bio-based coatings as potential barriers to chemical contaminants from recycled paper and board for food packaging. Food Addit Contam Part A 31(3):402–413. doi:10.1080/19440049.2013.86936

Kirwan MJ (2011) Paper and paperboard packaging. In: Coles R, Kirwan MJ (eds) Food and beverage packaging technology. Wiley-Blackwell, New York

Lee DS, Yam KL, Piergiovanni L (2008) Cellulose packaging. In: Lee DS, Yam KL, Piergiovanni L (eds) Food packaging science and technology. CRC Press, Boca Raton

Li F, Mascheroni E, Piergiovanni L (2015) The potential of nanocellulose in the packaging field: a review. Packag Technol Sci 28(6):475–564. doi:10.1002/pts.2121

Meyabadi TF, Dadashian F (2012) Optimization of enzymatic hydrolysis of waste cotton fibers for nanoparticles production using response surface methodology. Fiber Polym 13(3):313–321. doi:10.1007/s12221-012-0313-7

Piergiovanni L (2009) Packaging in the European Union. In: Yam KL (ed) The Wiley encyclopedia of packaging technology, 3rd edn. Wiley, Hoboken, pp 883–884

Roy D, Semsarilar M, Guthrie JT, Perrier S (2009) Cellulose modification by polymer grafting: a review. Chem Soc Rev 38(7):2046–2064. doi:10.1039/B808639G

Staudinger H (1926) Die Chemie der organischen hochmolekularen Stoffe im Sinne der Kekuléschen Strukturlehre. Ber Dtsch Chem Ges 59(12):3019–3043. doi:10.1002/cber.19260591206

Yam KL (ed) (2009) The Wiley Encyclopedia of Packaging Technology, 3rd edn. Wiley, Hoboken, p 910

Chapter 5
Plastic Packaging Materials

Abstract Words 'plastics' and 'polymers' are used quite often, particularly in the packaging sector, as synonymous even if they do not have the same meaning. These macromolecules are composed of many repeated subunits, i.e. definitely polymers. Actually, plastic packaging materials are predominately constituted of polymers (70–99 %) containing always various amounts of additives, such as plasticisers, antioxidants, pigments, antistatic, fillers and many other compounds. These chemicals are essential to provide the expected functionality; for this reason, final products are not definitely polymers. When speaking of food packaging applications, all starting substances, as well as finished plastics materials must have regulatory approvals, based on their specific chemical and toxicological features. Hereafter, the chemistry and general information about food packaging polymers are discussed here regarding two arbitrary categories: synthetic-oil derived polymers—polypropylene, polystyrene, polyvinyl chloride, etc.—on the one hand, and oil-derived and biodegradable bioplastics on the other side.

Keywords Addiction · Additives · Bioplastics · Bisphenol A · Condensation · Plasticisers · Plastics · Polymers

Abbreviations

PBSA	Aliphatic copolyester
PBAT	Aromatic co-polyester
BPA	Bisphenol A
PDLA	D-polylactic acid
EVA	Ethylene vinyl acetate copolymer
EVOH	Ethylene vinyl alcohol
EPS	Expanded polystyrene
XPS	Extruded polystyrene
PETG	Glycol-modified polyethylene terephthalate
HDPE	High density polyethylene
LLDPE	Linear low density polyethylene
LDPE	Low density polyethylene
PLLA	L-polylactic acid

MW	Molecular weight
MWD	Molecular weight distribution
OPET	Oriented polyethylene terephthalate
OPP	Oriented polypropylene
PHB	Poly-3- and poly-4-hydroxybutyrates
PCL	Polycaprolactone
PC	Polycarbonate
PET	Polyethylene Terephthalate
PHA	Polyhydroxyalkanoate
PLA	Polylactic acid
PDI	Polymer dispersity index
PP	Polypropylene
PS	Polystyrene
PVOH	Polyvinyl alcohol
PVC	Polyvinyl chloride
PVDC	Polyvinylidene chloride

5.1 Plastic Packaging Materials: An Overview

Words 'plastics' and 'polymers' are used quite often, particularly in the packaging sector, as synonymous even if they do not have the same meaning. In fact, not all the polymers can find useful packaging applications or exhibit plastic properties like, for example, chitin, proteins and nucleic acids. These macromolecules are composed of many repeated subunits, i.e. definitely polymers. Actually, plastic packaging materials are predominately constituted of polymers (70–99 %) containing always various amounts of additives, such as plasticisers, antioxidants, pigments, antistatic, fillers and many other compounds. These chemicals are essential to provide the expected functionality; for this reason, final products are not definitely polymers.

All the starting substances (monomers, additive, technological aids, etc.), as well as finished plastics materials, must have regulatory approvals for food contact applications, based on their specific chemical and toxicological features. Hereafter, the chemistry and general information about food packaging polymers are discussed here regarding two arbitrary categories: synthetic-oil derived polymers and bioplastics. No mention will be reserved to functional additives and to processes used to manufacture plastic packaging materials, because beyond the scope of this book.

5.2 Oil Derived Polymers

Polymers have quite different characteristics from smaller molecules: these peculiar properties (mechanical, barrier, optical and other features) rely on some factors which are both chemical and physical.

5.2.1 Molecular Weight

Synthetic polymers used in the manufacturing of plastic packaging materials have molecular weights (MW) typically between 50 and 200 kDa; these values are generally consistent with processing requirements (conversion in films; shaping process into final containers). Polymer MW significantly affect various physical properties; for instance, as MW raises, tensile and impact strengths sharply increase then slowly level off, while melt viscosity first increases gradually, and then sharply accelerates. A polymer has very rarely a single MW because molecules of different sizes are formed during the polymerisation process. Therefore, molecular weights distribution (MWD) and polymer dispersity index (PDI) can be quantified as measures of the frequency of polymer chains with different lengths (Holding and Meehan 1995). A broad MWD, for instance, tends to decrease tensile and impact strengths, increasing the processability because smaller molecules can act as plasticiser agents.

5.2.2 Intermolecular Forces

Intermolecular forces are responsible for holding together adjacent molecules: they range from weak dispersion forces to strong dipole-dipole interactions, depending on the chemical structure of molecules. Summation of intermolecular forces is particularly significant for polymer molecules due to their long chains; it can significantly influence mechanical, thermal, rheological features, and other properties of finished products. For some polymers, it is generally possible to influence their intermolecular forces, acting with the high energy provided by ionising radiations which may lead to some extent of cross linking (Nielsen 1969).

5.2.3 Chain Entanglement

The so-called 'chain entanglement' is the ability of a polymer chain to get entangled with another one; as a result, the length of polymer molecules increases. Chain entanglement holds polymer chains together, particularly at low temperature, making the complex polymer strong and resilient. At the same time, chains are allowed to slide each other at higher temperatures: this phenomenon permits poly-mers to be moulded into a finished container or in a film (thermoplastic behaviour).

5.2.4 Polymer Morphology

Polymer morphology corresponds to the arrangement of polymer molecules, leading to distinguishable regions (amorphous or crystalline) that can be detected by means of analytical techniques, such as scanning electron microscopy, X-ray diffraction or indirectly, differential scanning calorimetry. The chemical composi-tion, processing conditions and the cooling rate of molten polymers strongly affect the development of polymer morphology. When cooling time is prolonged, poly-mer chains can align into a pattern of crystalline region, as crystallinity may be defined as the presence of three-dimensional order on atomic dimensions level. Synthetic polymers used in plastic packaging materials have either amorphous or semi-crystalline structures (Fig. 5.1). Semi-crystalline morphology is often desir-able for final uses because it combines the strength of crystalline regions with the flexibility of amorphous regions. Amorphous and semi-crystalline polymers have different properties (Table 5.1) which may determine their final applications; it is worthy to underline that the crystallinity level can be changed during the manu-facturing of resins and finished products.

5.2.5 Molecular Orientation

Semi-crystalline polymers, in particular, are able to take great advantages from the orientation process. This procedure involves the stretching of polymeric chains below the melting temperature of polymers but above its glass-transition

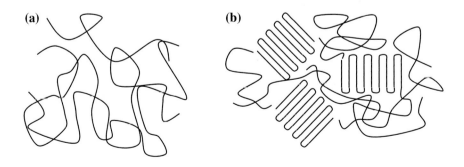

(a)   **(b)**

Amorphous polymer   Semi-crystalline polymer

Fig. 5.1 Amorphous (**a**) or semi-crystalline (**b**) structures typically present in synthetic polymers

Table 5.1 Properties of amorphous and semi-crystalline polymers (Hernandez 2009; Lee et al. 2008)

Semi-crystalline polymers	Isotropic (amorphous) polymers
The coexistence of crystalline and noncrystalline regions may be observed	Glassy below glass-transition temperature, similar to rubbers (elastic, soft) above this thermal value
Because of the peculiar transmission of light, crystalline regions can give a visual appearance from cloudy to opaque	Clear in appearance
Specific melting temperature, or a range of melting thermal values	No melting temperature
These products can be quite strong and brittle. On the other hand impact resistance performances are reduced if compared with other polymers	They can be quite weak and flexible
Gas barrier effect: moderate to good performances	Gas barrier effect: poor to moderate performances
Good performances against chemical agents	Moderate resistance to chemical agents
General properties are strongly influenced by cooling rate and orientation	General properties are substantially unaffected or moderately influenced by cooling rate and orientation

temperature. Usually, the molecular orientation can be given during blown film extrusion, injection stretch blow moulding, and in a tenter frame after cast film extrusion. The orientation can be forced either uniaxially or biaxially (in both machine and transverse directions), leading to mono- or bi-oriented packages. The consequent alignment of polymer chains and modifications in polymer morphology can lead to important improvements of optical, mechanical and barrier properties. Moreover, oriented films have the predisposition to shrink with heating, making available shrink packaging.

5.2.6 Tacticity

According to the International Union of Pure and Applied Chemistry (Jenkins et al. 1996), tacticity is defined as 'the orderliness of the succession of configurational repeating units in the main chain of a regular macromolecule'. Tacticity can significantly affect many physical properties of polymers and consequently possible useful applications. In particular, vinyl polymers of the type: $-[CH(R)-H_2C]-$, can show three types of alignment: each repeating unit with substituent R on the one side of the polymer backbone, is followed by the next monomer with R substituent on the same side (isotactic type), the other side as the previous one (syndiotactic polymer) or they are positioned randomly (atactic type).

Polypropylene, polyvinyl chloride and polystyrene are typical vinyl polymers, quite used in food packaging: they show tacticity (Fig. 5.2) and many important properties of the atactic type are hugely different than isotactic types, in particular for PP. Up to the proposal of Ziegler-Natta catalysis in the 1960s (Sinn and Kaminsky 1980), only the atactic form was synthesised with no useful applications, while nowadays PP is produced as isotactic semi-crystalline polymer. PP is now the second polymer used in food packaging, accounting for 1/5 of the total plastics mass.

5.2.7   Polymers for Food Packaging. Main Features

In the following Sections, a synthetic description of the main characteristics of most common polymers for plastic packaging production is discussed. They are listed in order of importance, from the most abundant (about 50 %) polyethylene, to minor polymers that all together account for less than 2 % of the total mass of plastics for food packaging purposes. The basic formulas of discussed polymers are reported in Fig. 5.2, while the meaning of all symbols used for plastic polymers used in packaging is reported together in Fig. 5.3 with related codes for recycling purposes.

5.2.7.1   Polyethylene (PE)

Ethylene, the simplest alkene (olefin), can polymerise by the addition mechanism (also known as chain-growth polymerisation), in which monomers are covalently linked together into long chains, thanks to the double bond in the molecule (electrophilic addition).

The process needs an initiator able to form a reactive radical onto unsaturated monomers; then the reactive intermediate can add to other monomers without formation of any by-product. Depending on polymerisation conditions (pressure and temperature) and used catalysts, morphology and density of produced PE may be deeply modified.

The most common polyethylene types used in food packaging are high density polyethylene (HDPE), low density polyethylene (LDPE), and linear low density polyethylene (LLDPE). They are different in density, chain branching, crystallinity and consequently, in mechanical, optical and barrier properties. HDPE is a linear polymer with few side-chain branches, strong and not clear (hazy) for its high crystallinity. Compared to LDPE, HDPE has better chemical resistance, a higher melting point (typically 135 °C vs. 110 °C), greater tensile strength and hardness. LDPE has many side-chain branches; it is soft, flexible and stretchable. In addition, it has good clarity and heat sealability. Hence, LDPE is almost always the inner layer of multilayer structures with another option: it can be also used as adhesive in extrusion coating steps of production.

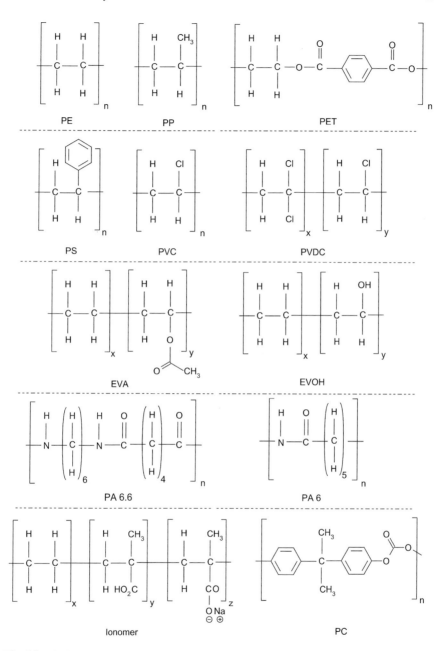

Fig. 5.2 The basic formulas of polymers commonly used in packaging applications: polyethylene (*PE*); polypropylene (*PP*); polyethylene terephthalate (*PET*); polystyrene (*PS*); polyvinyl chloride (*PVC*); polyvinylidene chloride (*PVDC*); ethylene vinyl acetate copolymer (*EVA*); ethylene vinyl alcohol copolymer (*EVOH*); polyamides 6.6 (*PA 6.6*); polyamides 6 (*PA 6*); ionomers; polycarbonate (*PC*). BKchem version 0.13.0, 2009 (http://bkchem.zirael.org/index.html) has been used for drawing these structures

Fig. 5.3 Symbols for plastic
materials

Poly(ethylene terephthalate)

High density polyethylene

Poly(vinyl chloride)

Low density poly(ethylene)
Linear low density poly(ethylene)

Poly(propylene)
Oriented poly(propylene)

Poly(styrene)
High Impact Poly(styrene)
Expanded Poly(styrene)

Poly(amide)

Poly(amide) 6

Poly(amide) 6,6

Poly(amide) 12

Poly(carbonate)

Poly(vinylidene chloride)

Ethylen vinyl alcohol

Ethylen vinyl acetate

Poly(tetrafluoroethylene)

Perfluoroalkoxy alkanes

Fluorinated ethylene propylene

LLDPE is a copolymer having 1–10 % of other alkene co-monomers. The
co-monomer presence leads to long and linear chains with many short side-chain
branches. It has similar clarity and heat sealability as LDPE and the strength and
toughness of HDPE. Recently, many developments in controlling the

polymerisation process (single-site or metallocene catalysis) allow to produce LLPDE films with superior thermal, optical and mechanical properties.

5.2.7.2 Polypropylene (PP)

PP has high crystallinity, but a very low density (0.9 g cm^{-3}) and good clearness, due to the helical shape of its isotactic structure (Meille et al. 1994). Compared to PE, PP has higher tensile strength, stiffness, hardness and a higher melting temperature (165 °C). PP films are available both in oriented, either uniaxially or biaxially, and in non-oriented forms; oriented polypropylene (OPP) films have significantly improved strength, stiffness and gas barrier, but these materials are not heat-sealable. PP and OPP films are the main polypropylene applications; they can also be very important when speaking of injection moulded and thermoformed containers and closures.

5.2.7.3 Polyethylene Terephthalate (PET)

As all polyesters, PET—the most important one for this chemical group in packaging—is obtained by condensation polymerisation, a form of step-growth polymerisation. In this particular process two molecules join through the liberation of water (in other situations, small molecules). Using monomers with two reactive ends (e.g. di-alcohols and bi-carboxylic acids), linear polyesters are mainly created, while monomers with more than two end groups give three-dimensional, cross-linked polymers. Polyethylene terephthalate, a semi-crystalline polymer, can be transformed in final products which have amorphous structure (amorphous PET), thus very transparent, or crystallised (crystallised PET), opaque and more heat resistant. They can be turned into films, trays or bottles, both biaxially oriented and non-oriented. Often, various co-monomers are used in the polymerisation in order to modify some properties. Glycol-modified polyethylene terephthalate (PETG) is the most common modification in the packaging sector; PETG has higher stiffness, hardness, and toughness as well as better impact strength than PET.

5.2.7.4 Polystyrene (PS)

PS is an amorphous, very clear polymer, commonly in the atactic form. However, a syndiotactic, crystallised PS can be also produced. Typical properties of the amorphous polymer are low gas barrier, intermediate water vapour barrier, hardness, and quite low impact strength (consequently, PS is a fragile material). A high-impact PS is also available as a blend of polystyrene, polybutadiene, and grafted polystyrene-polybutadiene copolymer. PS has relatively low melting point (88 °C); consequently, it has also high processability that allows it to be easily thermoformed or injection moulded into various containers (cups, closures, and dishware). Various important applications of PS are in the expanded forms: expanded polystyrene (EPS) and extruded polystyrene (XPS), in which the original density (0.96–1.04 g cm^{-3}) is brought to quite low values of bulk densities such as 0.01–01.45 g cm^{-3}. EPS is made of pre-expanded polystyrene beads, while XPS foam is manufactured by adding foaming agents directly in the extrusion process.

5.2.7.5   Polyvinyl Chloride (PVC)

PVC is the least 'organic' among plastic packaging materials, because more than 56 % of its MW is due to inorganic chloride. Polyvinyl chloride is produced by polymerisation of the vinyl chloride monomer, which is, in turn, obtained by ethylene chlorination. The monomer has been recognised as a powerful human carcinogen substance mainly by inhalation and its residual content in the polymer is carefully checked. The clear, atactic, amorphous polymer is rigid and shows poor thermal processing stability. Therefore, PVC is most often added with plasticisers to achieve widely varying properties, depending on the type and amount of added plasticisers. Safety concerns have been raised about the possible migration of monomeric plasticisers (e.g. diethylhexyl adipate, diethylhexyl phthalate), in particular from plasticised PVC 'cling' film. PVC has a very good processability: various different kinds of packages can be easily produced by thermoforming and blow moulding techniques.

5.2.7.6   Polyamide (PA)

Polyamides belong to a family of polymers obtained by condensation of monomers: di-amines and bi-carboxylic acids, or amino acids that have both functional ends in the same molecule. The final aim is to provide the amide group. One or two numbers are used beside the PA symbol to indicate the chain length of used monomers. Therefore, 'PA 6.6' is the polyamide obtained by adipic acid and hexamethylenediamine, while 'PA 6' is the polyamide obtained by 6-aminohexanoic (6-caproic acid), in particular from its lactam (cyclic amide) ε-caprolactam. These polymers are the two most common PA for food packaging films, very often still named with the original brand name 'Nylon' by DuPont.

PA properties can vary in a broad range, according to its MW and crystallinity; in general, these polymers have good gas barrier, puncture resistance, and heat resistance properties. Moreover, some aromatic PA, such as polymetaxylylene adipamide from aromatic monomers, are known; however, they find few applications in the packaging sector.

5.2.7.7 Minor Polymers

Polyvinylidene chloride (PVDC), a copolymer of vinylidene chloride (85–90 %) and vinyl chloride, is commercialised under the trade name 'Saran'. It is mostly used in multilayer films and containers coating. Unlike PVC , PVDC cannot present a tacticity because of the symmetry of its monomer. The first use of Saran has been reported in the '50s as functional coating for cellophane, providing moisture barrier and heat sealability to regenerated cellulose films. Actually, the most notable advantages of PVDC are related to its excellent oxygen and moisture barriers.

Another, more important, copolymer is ethylene vinyl alcohol (EVOH) which also has very good performance as oxygen barrier; in addition, it is much more common in multilayer structures, nowadays. Depending on molar proportions of ethylene and vinyl alcohol in the copolymer, barrier properties can change hugely. Oxygen barrier is reduced when ethylene content increases; on the other side, moisture sensitivity increases while increasing the vinyl component or moisture resistance decreases while increasing the vinyl component; finally, oxygen barrier increases as well as the water sensitivity. EVOH is generally used with ethylene concentration around 32 % and it is not obtained through direct polymerisation: the process is the hydrolysis of the corresponding ester, ethylene vinyl acetate copolymer (EVA). This is a totally different material with any oxygen barrier properties: it can be very interesting if used as heat seal layers for various kinds of packages.

More importantly, EVA copolymers are the most used polymers for hot-melt manufacturing, due to their high versatility in formulations. Among the polymers relevant for their adhesive properties and heat sealing functionality, 'ionomers' deserve to be mentioned.

Ionomers are polymers containing small portions of ionic units; they are generally based on ethylene and methacrylic acid copolymers. Methacrylic acid groups, typically less than 15 % of the polymer molecule, are partially neutralised by sodium, zinc or other metallic cations. The simultaneous presence of nonpolar ethylene groups, polar methacrylic acid groups and carboxylate ionic pairs provide the ionomer with an original combination of properties. Possible ionic crosslinks among polymer chains are reversible, unlike covalent crosslinks; forces of the ionic crosslinks are greatly reduced when the ionomer is heated, allowing the free movement of polymer chains. Therefore, sealing and formability are excellent performances of flexible packaging materials that include ionomers.

Polycarbonate (PC) is the amorphous polyester obtained by transesterification from bisphenol A (BPA) and diphenyl carbonate. PC is a very clear and tough polymer that allows the production of light and infrangible alternatives to glass containers by injection-moulding, blow moulding, or thermoforming techniques. Further, PC may be considered as an ovenable material because it withstands temperatures above 200 °C. Currently, there is a big concern about the possible migration of BPA, which is believed an endocrine disruptor, in particular for its large use in baby bottles manufacturing (Shelnutt et al. 2013).

5.3 Bioplastics

The word 'bioplastics' refers to a family of materials with quite different characteristics; it has recently received a clear (but quite often un-properly used) definition by the European Bioplastics Organization (Anonymous 2013). A material is defined as a bioplastic if it is either bio-based, biodegradable, or shows both these two properties. Therefore, bioplastics correspond to three main groups of different materials:

(1) Bio-based, or partially bio-based, non-biodegradable plastics, such as polyethylene (bio-PE), polypropylene (bio-PP), polyvinyl chloride (bio-PVC) or polyester (bio-PET), that are synthetised starting from bio-based raw materials but identical to current polymers based on fossil resources and above described
(2) Plastics that are both bio-based and biodegradable, such as polylactic acid (PLA) or polyhydroxyalkanoate (PHA), described in the following Sections
(3) Plastics that are obtained starting from oil products. Because of their MW and intrinsic characteristics, they are biodegradable. Examples: aromatic co-polyesters (PBAT), aliphatic copolyesters (PBSA), polycaprolactone (PCL), thermoplastic polyvinyl alcohol (PVOH). These substances are also shortly presented further.

The classification shows and underlines that biodegradability depends on the chemical composition, not on the origin of a material (Sect. 7.2). It also enlightens the debate currently ongoing about the opportunity of biodegradable materials for food packaging. Quite obviously, the replacement of petrochemical carbon with biological carbon in a packaging material is a good way to reduce its carbon footprint at values close to zero (Narayan 2012) and might make the packaging biodegradable. However, biodegradability is not unanimously considered as the best choice for a single-use package; according to many authors (Robertson 2014), the conversion of a solid material into gases (by composting and/or biodegradation) should be considered as a last resort, preferring the capture of the embodied energy and material mass for reuse through recycling or the recovering of energy content through incineration. In particular, composting or biodegradation of a bio-based material seems a wasteful approach: these choices may even enhance and load the collection of food-contaminated packaging instead of reducing the landfill volume.

Another issue coming from this nomenclature concerns how to estimate how much bio-based is a bioplastic. A unique procedure or a generally accepted global standard does not exist yet, but bio-based bioplastics can be described by their 'bio-based carbon content' or 'bio-based mass content'. The European Committee for Standardization (CEN) has published a technical specification in 2006 with relation to the determination of biogenic carbon content in solid recovered fuels (CEN/TS 15440:2006). More recently, ASTM also has published a standard to measure the bio-based carbon content using radiocarbon analysis (ASTM 2012).

5.3.1 Polylactic Acid (PLA)

PLA is generally considered as the bioplastic material with best chances of development; in fact, it has already many applications in food packaging (Siracusa et al. 2012). PLA is chemically synthetised starting from simple sugars obtained from biomass and fermented to lactic acid (Garlotta 2001). Because of the chiral nature of lactic acid, two enantiomers—L- and D-polylactic acids (PLLA, PDLA) —exist. As a result, three different polymers are available: PLLA, PDLA and the most common mixture of the two which shows the maximum crystallinity for the nucleating effect provided by PDLA.

Two main routes are known to produce PLA starting from lactic acid or from the cyclic di-ester, lactide (Mehta et al. 2005; Cheng et al. 2009). The most common is the ring opening polymerisation of lactide with various metal catalysts (typically tin octoate). Using lactic acid monomers, the polymerisation takes place by their direct condensation with the elimination of a water molecule at high temperature but less than 200 °C, with the consequent lactide monomer formation instead of poly-merisation. Anyway, water generation is undesirable because leads to low MW-materials. A common issue of all PLA polymers is their tendency to degrade for hydrolysis phenomena, transesterification interchains with lactide formation and oxidative breakage; all these reactions are promoted and fastened by temperature, acidic pH values and small contaminants.

Generally speaking, the properties of PLA are interesting for food packaging but not totally satisfying so far. PLA-oxygen barrier values are intermediate between PET and PS while water vapour permeability is similar to the PA6 polyamide.

5.3.2 Polyhydroxyalkanoate (PHA)

Linear polyesters, named PHA, constitute a family of both bio-based and biosyn-thetised bioplastics produced by the bacteria *Cupriavidus necator* (originally known as *Alcaligenes eutrophus* and then *Ralstonia eutropha*) through the fer-mentation of sugars (e.g. glucose or sucrose) or lipids (e.g. vegetable oil or glyc-erine). From intracellular inclusions (highly refractive granules), PHA may be extracted up to 80 % of the microorganism dry weight. Their biosynthesis is usually due to lack of macro-elements (such as phosphorus, nitrogen, trace elements or oxygen) and to the excess of carbon sources.

More than 150 different monomers have been found in this heterogeneous family of homo or copolyesters, having very different properties (Doi and Steinbüchel 2002) and leading to either thermoplastic or elastomeric materials, with melting temperatures ranging from 40 to 180 °C.

The most common PHA is poly-3-hydroxybutyrate, but also poly-4-hydroxybutyrate and polyhydroxyvalerate are quite used. PHA differs in their properties according to their chemical composition, but in general they show low water vapour permeability with a crystallinity in the range of a few to 70 %. Poly-3- and poly-4-hydroxybutyrates (PHB) properties are similar to polypropylene, having good resistance to moisture and aroma barrier properties. On the other hand, PHB are relatively brittle and stiff. However, PHB copolymers with fatty acids such as beta-hydroxyvalerateacid may be even elastic.

5.3.3   Starch Polymers

Different companies—Novamont in Italy, Plantic in Australia, Biotec-Sphere, Roquette, Limagrain in France and Cereplast in USA—have developed bio-based and biodegradable new materials, based on gelatinized starches (Mohammadi et al. 2013; Xie et al. 2012; Halley and Avérous 2014), often in combination with other biologically and non-biologically sourced polymers.

At present, one of the most developed and used starch polymers is Mater-Bi® from Novamont (Bastioli 1998). The 'Mater-Bi®' brand name refers to a broad family of bioplastics obtained by the combination, with proprietary technologies, of starch, cellulose and vegetable oils. Their most common use of this product is correlated with bags for separate waste collection, but the polymer can also find application in the food service, large-scale retail distribution, personal care, packaging and agriculture. Many different types of bio-based polymers like Mater-Bi® are available at present. Generally, they can contain or not starch; other possible biodegradable polymers may be obtained from renewable or fossil-derived sources. Starch-based polymers present highly diversified structures in which the starch either forms a complex with other polymer components or presents a very fine dispersed morphology, which makes the products particularly tough. Because of the necessity of improving technical features and economic interests, some special polyesters can be obtained from vegetable oils: an example is the brand Origo-Bi® (Novamont). Properties of these bioplastics vary considerably as regards their mechanical properties and transparency but all the grades are certified according to European and international standards with regard to their biodegradability in various disposal environments.

5.3.4   Oil-Derived and Biodegradable Bioplastics

Few synthetic polymers, obtained from petrochemical sources, show a complete biodegradability in different environments for their specific characteristics. Their use in packaging application is limited up to now because of their price, with the exception of polyvinyl alcohol. Actually, polyvinyl alcohol is used more for its outstanding oxygen barrier properties than for its biodegradability.

5.3.4.1 Aromatic and Aliphatic Co-polyesters

Typically, biodegradable polyesters (PBAT, PBSA) contain a high fraction of aliphatic ester groups because aromatic dicarboxylic acids are much less sensitive to hydrolysis than aliphatic polyesters (Chen et al. 2008). Aromatic and aliphatic copolyesters, combining the biodegradability of aliphatic polyesters with the physical properties of aromatic polyesters, may have interesting perspectives also in packaging applications.

5.3.4.2 Polycaprolactone

PCL is prepared by ring opening polymerisation of ε-caprolactone using a catalyst, typically tin octoate (Fig. 5.4). Recently, a wide range of catalysts for the ring opening polymerisation of caprolactone have been reviewed (Labet and Thielemans 2009).

PCL is degraded via hydrolysis of its ester bonds in various conditions; therefore, it has received a great attention for use as an implantable biomaterial and as packaging material as well. Recently, PCL has been considered in the potential development of active packaging with enhanced barrier properties and controlled-release of thymol, a very effective natural antimicrobial (Sanchez-Garcia et al. 2008).

5.3.4.3 Polyvinyl Alcohol (PVOH)

Differently from other vinyl polymers, PVOH is not prepared by polymerisation of the corresponding monomer. In fact, this monomer—vinyl alcohol—is unstable due to keto–enol tautomerism: i.e. a chemical equilibrium between a keto form (in this case acetaldehyde) and an enol one (vinyl alcohol). Polyvinyl alcohol is therefore prepared by first polymerising vinyl acetate, and the resulting polyvinyl acetate is converted to PVOH (Hallensleben 2000).

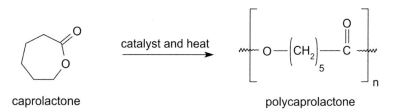

caprolactone   polycaprolactone

Fig. 5.4 A scheme of polycaprolactone (*PCL*) production, via ring opening polymerisation of ε-caprolactone. BKchem version 0.13.0, 2009 (http://bkchem.zirael.org/index.html) has been used for drawing this structure

polyvinyl acetate   polyvinyl alcohol

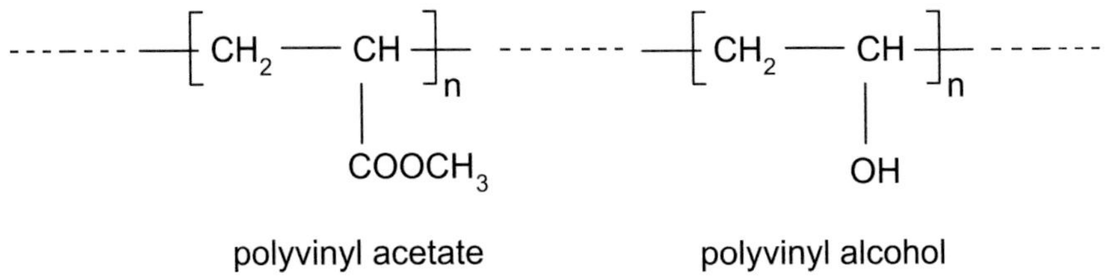

Fig. 5.5 A synthetic but biodegradable polyvinyl acetate/polyvinyl alcohol copolymer. BKchem version 0.13.0, 2009 (http://bkchem.zirael.org/index.html) has been used for drawing this structure

The conversion of polyester is usually conducted by base-catalysed transesterification with ethanol and some acetate is often present, affecting final properties (Fig. 5.5). The worldwide consumption of PVOH is quite high: over one million metric tons (Chinn et al. 2007) because of its application in different fields.

As already stated, the use of PVOH in the packaging sector is mainly related to the production of very high oxygen barriers. Polyvinyl alcohol is perfectly water-soluble and is recognised as one of the very few vinyl polymers susceptible of ultimate biodegradation in the presence of suitably microorganisms (Amann and Minge 2012; Chiellini et al. 2003; Xanthos 2005).

References

Amann M, Minge O (2012) Biodegradability of Poly(vinyl acetate) and related polymers. In: Rieger B, Künkel A, Coates GW, Reichardt R, Dinjus E, Zevaco TA (eds) Synthetic biodegradable polymers. Adv Polym Sci 245:137–172. Springer, Berlin. doi:10.1007/12_2011_153

Anonymous (2013) Bioplastics—facts and figures. European Bioplastics e.V., Berlin. http://en.european-bioplastics.org/wp-content/uploads/2013/publications/EuBP_FactsFigures_bioplastics_2013.pdf. Accessed 29 May 2015

ASTM (2012) Active Standard ASTM D6866-12—Standard test methods for determining the biobased content of solid, liquid, and gaseous samples using radiocarbon analysis, ASTM Volume 08.03 Plastics (III): D5117 latest; Reinforced plastic piping systems and chemical equipment; Plastic building products. ASTM International, West Conshohocken. doi:10.1520/D6866-12

Bastioli C (1998) Properties and applications of Mater-Bi starch-based materials. Polym Degrad Stab 59(1–3):263–272. doi:10.1016/S0141-3910(97)00156-0

Chen Y, Tan L, Chen L, Yang Y, Wang X (2008) Study on biodegradable aromatic/aliphatic copolyesters. Brazil J Chem Eng 25:321–335. doi:10.1590/S0104-66322008000200011

Cheng Y, Deng S, Chen P, Ruan R (2009) Polylactic acid (PLA) synthesis and modifications: a review. Front Chem China 4(3):259–264. doi:10.1007/s11458-009-0092-x

Chiellini E, Corti A, D'Antone S, Solaro R (2003) Biodegradation of poly (vinyl alcohol) based materials. Prog Polym Sci 28(6):963–1014. doi:http://dx.doi.org/10.1016/S0079-6700(02)00149-1

Chinn H, Inoguchi Y, Loechner U (2007) SRI consulting CEH report polyvinyl alcohol. SRI Consulting, Menlo Park

Doi Y, Steinbüchel A (2002) Biopolymers, polyesters III-applications and commercial products, vol 4. Wiley-Blackwell, New York

Garlotta D (2001) A literature review of poly(lactic acid). J Polym Environ 9(2):63–84. doi:10.1023/A:1020200822435

Hallensleben ML (2000) Polyvinyl compounds, others. In: Elvers B (ed) Ullmann's encyclopedia of industrial chemistry. Wiley-VCH Verlag GmbH & Co. KGaA, Weinheim. doi:10.1002/14356007.a21_743

Halley P, Avérous L (eds) (2014) Starch polymers: from genetic engineering to green applications. Elsevier B.V, Amsterdam

Hernandez RJ (2009) Polymer properties. In: Yam KL (ed) The Wiley encyclopedia of packaging technology, 3rd edn. Wiley, New York

Holding SR, Meehan E (1995) Molecular weight characterisation of synthetic polymers. Rapra Technology Limited, Telford

Jenkins AD, Kratochvíl P, Stepto RFT, Suter UW (1996) Glossary of basic terms in polymer science (IUPAC Recommendations 1996). Pure Appl Chem 68(12):2287–2311. doi:10.1351/pac199668122287

Labet M, Thielemans W (2009) Synthesis of polycaprolactone: a review. Chem Soc Rev 38(12):3484–3504. doi:10.1039/B820162P

Lee DS, Yam KL, Piergiovanni L (2008) Food packaging polymers. In: Lee DS, Yam KL, Piergiovanni L (eds) Food packaging science and technology. CRC Press, Boca Raton

Mehta R, Kumar V, Bhunia H, Upadhyay SN (2005) Synthesis of poly(lactic acid): a review. J Macromol Sci Part C 45(4):325–349. doi:10.1080/15321790500304148

Meille SV, Ferro DR, Brueckner S, Lovinger AJ, Padden FJ (1994) Structure of .beta.-isotactic polypropylene: a long-standing structural puzzle. Macromol 27(9):2615–2622. doi:10.1021/ma00087a034

Mohammadi Nafchi A, Moradpour M, Saeidi M, Alias AK (2013) Thermoplastic starches: properties, challenges, and prospects. Starch - Stärke 65(1–2):61–72. doi:10.1002/star.201200201

Narayan R (2012) Biobased and biodegradable plastics: rationale, drivers, and technology exemplars. In: Khemani K, Scholz C (eds) Degradable polymers and materials: principles and practice, 2nd edn. ACS Symposium Series, American Chemical Society, Washington, DC, pp 13–31. doi:10.1021/bk-2012-1114.ch002

Nielsen LE (1969) Cross-linking–effect on physical properties of polymers. J Macromol Sci Part C 3(1):69–103. doi:10.1080/15583726908545897

Robertson GL (2014) Biobased but not biodegradable. Food Technol 68(6):61–70

Sanchez-Garcia MD, Ocio MJ, Gimenez E, Lagaron JM (2008) Novel polycaprolactone nanocomposites containing thymol of interest in antimicrobial film and coating applications. J Plast Film Sh 24(3–4):239–251. doi:10.1177/8756087908101539

Shelnutt S, Kind J, Allaben W (2013) Bisphenol A: update on newly developed data and how they address NTP's 2008 finding of 'Some Concern'. Food Chem Toxicol 57:284–295. doi:10.1016/j.fct.2013.03.027

Sinn H, Kaminsky W (1980) Ziegler-Natta catalysis. Adv Organometal Chem 18:99–149. doi:10.1016/S0065-3055(08)60307-X

Siracusa V, Blanco I, Romani S, Tylewicz U, Rocculi P, Rosa MD (2012) Poly(lactic acid)-modified films for food packaging application: physical, mechanical, and barrier behavior. J Appl Polymer Sci 125(S2):E390–E401. doi:10.1002/app.36829

Xanthos M (2005) Polymers and polymer composites. In: Xanthos M (ed) Functional fillers for plastics. Wiley-VCH Verlag GmbH & Co. KGaA, Weinheim, pp 1–16

Xie F, Halley PJ, Avérous L (2012) Rheology to understand and optimize processibility, structures and properties of starch polymeric materials. Prog Polym Sci 37(4):595–623. doi:10.1016/j.progpolymsci.2011.07.002

Chapter 6
Materials Combinations

Abstract A single material is used rarely alone in the manufacturing of final packages, in particular when speaking of flexible packaging. Various materials can be used in order to assemble a structure with interesting properties (logistic advantages, ameliorated shelf lives of packaged products, opportunities for recycling and environmental impacts). This reflection should address more attention to the possible development of high-performing packages which can extend shelf lives and better protect foods. The most important technologies used to arrange together different materials in order to achieve more performing packages—multilayer structures, composites, polymer blends and alloys—are shortly described in this chapter with emphasis on chemical aspects.

Keywords Alloys · Blends · Coating · Coextrusion · Composites · Environmental impact · Lamination · Multilayer materials · Polymers · Recycling

Abbreviations

ACC	All-cellulose composite
α	Aspect ratio
CNCs	Cellulose nanocrystals
EMAA	Ethylene-methacrylic acid
EVA	Ethylene vinyl acetate copolymer
EVOH	Ethylene vinyl alcohol
GWP	Global warming potential
HDPE	High-density polyethylene
HIPS	High-impact polystyrene
IUPAC	International Union of Pure and Applied Chemistry
LDPE	Low-density polyethylene
MEK	Methyl ethyl ketone
OPA	Oriented polyamide
OPP	Oriented polypropylene
PO_2	Oxygen permeability
PA	Polyamide
PET	Polyethylene Terephthalate

© The Author(s) 2016
L. Piergiovanni and S. Limbo, *Food Packaging Materials*,
Chemistry of Foods, DOI 10.1007/978-3-319-24732-8_6

PA/MXD 6   Poly(m-xylyleneadipamide)PA/MXD 6
PP   Polypropylene
PU   Polyurethane
PVOH   Polyvinyl alcohol
PVDC   Polyvinylidene chloride
PAA   Primary aromatic amine
A/V   Surface area/volume
VOC   Volatile organic compound

6.1 Materials Combinations. An Overview

Very rarely, in particular for flexible packaging, a material alone is used in the manufacturing of final packages. More frequently, various materials are used in order to assemble a structure that can accomplish all the targets of containment and distribution and assure desired shelf lives of packaged foods or beverages. Therefore, the complexity of packaging is augmented from a chemical point of view; this argument is generally considered as a serious issue, as far as opportunities for recycling and environmental impacts are concerned. Doubtless, the more complex is the structure of a final material, the less easy are material recovery and recycling. However, one point should be clearly underlined concerning the general environmental impact of modern packages.

The most common indicator of environmental impact is usually considered to be the global warming potential (GWP), i.e. the total amount of greenhouse gases (carbon footprint) related to the production, use and disposal of a specific good. However, what is generally misunderstood is that GWP values of food products (production and processing) are 20–200 times higher than GWP of their corresponding packaging (Wikström and Williams 2010; Grönman et al. 2013). These figures, therefore, should address more attention to the possible development of high-performing packages, even if more complex, able to extend shelf lives and better protect foods. In fact, a reduction of food loss and waste by means of high-performing packages might be more sustainable for the environment and global sustainability (Silvenius et al. 2014). The most important technologies used to arrange together different materials in order to achieve more performing packages are shortly described in this chapter with emphasis on the chemical aspects.

6.2 Multilayers Materials

The industrial sector involved in converting packaging materials and manufacturing final packages has many processes and technologies to achieve targets. The most common processes to arrange multilayers structures are coextrusion (Mount 2010), adhesive lamination (Wagner 2010), coating (Gutoff and Cohen 2010), metallisation (Bishop and Mount 2010), multi-injection moulding and multilayered cardboards forming. All of them make it possible structures consisting of surfaces overlapping of different materials, i.e. multilayer structures. Many of these technologies allow the superimposition even of ten diverse layers, in few micrometres of total thickness.

6.2.1 Coextrusion

Coextrusion allows multilayer structures manufacturing of thermoplastic materials for various applications using two or more extruders and a unique extrusion die. A basic assumption to achieve successfully a coextrusion process is the chemical and thermal compatibility of overlapped thermoplastic polymers. The proximity of melting temperatures is essential, as well as flow properties at melting temperature, and chemical interactions between each layer. To overcome problems, coextrusion process might involve polymer compatibilisers or tie layers as intermediate layers. The general principle of compatibilisation is to reduce interfacial energy between two polymers in order to increase adhesion.

Coextrusion, possibly assisted by appropriate tie layers, is extensively used in the manufacturing of modern flexible packaging materials and is the leading technology for valorisation of recycled streams. Table 6.1 shows some examples of typical coextruded multilayer structures.

Moreover, coextruded sheets of adequate thickness may be conveniently thermoformed into trays or cups, leading to multilayer structures of three-dimensional packages.

Table 6.1 Examples of multilayers structure obtained by coextrusion

Multilayer structure	Application
High-impact polystyrene (HIPS)/adhesive/PVDC/HIPS	Thermoforming films and sheets
PP/adhesive/ethylene vinyl alcohol (EVOH)/adhesive/high density polyethylene (HDPE)	Retortable semi-rigid films and sheets
Virgin PET/recycled PET/virgin PET	Thermoforming films and sheets
PA/adhesive/LDPE	Flexible film
Low-density polyethylene (LDPE)/EVOH/LDPE	Flexible film
LDPE/PA/tie layer/EVOH/tie layer/PA/LDPE	Film, thermoforming sheets
PE/adhesive/EVOH/adhesive/HIPS	Thermoforming films and sheets

6.2.2   Adhesive Lamination

A totally different approach can be used in multilayers manufacturing starting from already available plan films or sheets, on condition that an adequate adhesive is used to join individual layers. The process is definitely much more versatile because whatever material (paper, board, aluminum foil) can be combined with whatever substrate, selecting properly the adhesive.

An important classification is related to the kind of used adhesive. Three main products—solvent-based, water-based and solventless-based (mono- and bicomponent) adhesives—are commonly available; a special case of lamination, named 'extrusion lamination', uses melted polymers as adhesive to join individual layers. A huge number of different options are known and a complete list of them is beyond the scope of this chapter. Only the main issues of different processes are mentioned here with special reference to the chemistry of adhesion.

Most used waterborne adhesives are polyurethane (PU), but also solvent-based PU are well established and used for packaging materials. Their chemistry is based on the polymerisation between a di-alcohol (or polyol) and a di-isocyanate (or polyisocyanate) that can be both, aliphatic or aromatic, synthetic or bio-based, leading to both thermoplastic or thermosetting polymers (Fig. 6.1).

Currently, a strong trend in food packaging is towards the use of water-based adhesives in order to avoid possible 'volatile organic compounds' (VOC) contamination from solvents, mainly methyl ethyl ketone (also named MEK), ethyl acetate, acetone, toluene and few others. Some taint problems, for instance, had arisen through the reaction of VOC such as mesityl oxide, which may be a common contaminant of acetone, with hydrogen sulphide that might be present in some protein foods. The result would be the adduct 4-methyl-4-mercaptopentan-2-one which has a very strong and bad off-flavour (Franz et al. 1990).

However, the main problem coming from PU adhesives is probably the potential migration of toxic primary aromatic amines (PAA) from residual aromatic isocyanates (Franz and Störmer 2008; de Poças-Fatima and Hogg 2007). Actually, isocyanate can hydrolyse reacting with water, with the consequent production of primary amines and carbon dioxide, according to the reaction in Fig. 6.2.

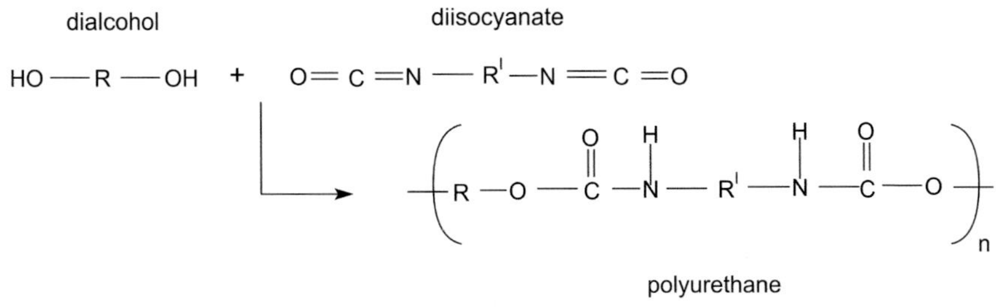

Fig. 6.1 The synthetic pathway for polyurethane polymerisation. BKchem version 0.13.0, 2009 (http://bkchem.zirael.org/index.html) has been used for drawing these structures

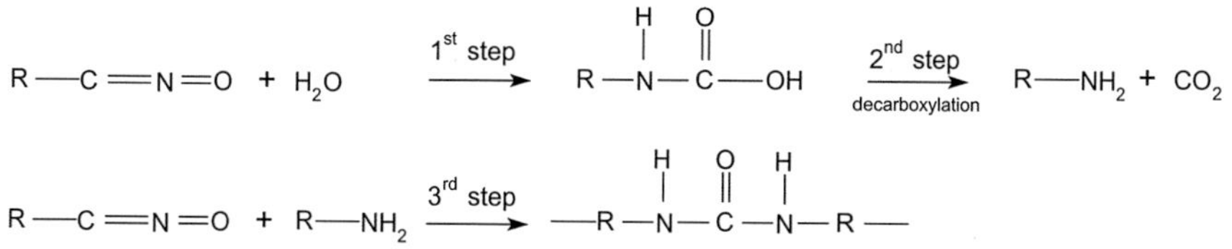

Fig. 6.2 The potential formation of toxic primary amines from isocyanate. BKchem version 0.13.0, 2009 (http://bkchem.zirael.org/index.html) has been used for drawing these structures

Table 6.2 Examples of multilayers structure obtained by lamination and application in food

Multilayer structure	Application
Oriented polypropylene (OPP)/adhesive/ethylene vinyl acetate copolymer (EVA)	Flexible film
OPP/coextruded polypropylene (PP)	Flexible film
OPP/adhesive/OPP/PVDC	Flexible film
Cellophane/adhesive/LDPE	Flexible film
PET/Aluminum/Peelable polymer blend	Peelable 'snap open' closure
Metallised PA/LDPE/EVA	Flexible film
PA/adhesive/EVA	Flexible film
OPP/PVDC/Ionomers	Flexible film
Paper/LDPE	Semi-rigid material
PE/Ink/Board/PE/aluminum foil/tie layer or primer/PE	Aseptic beverage carton

The moisture present in food can permeate the laminate and bring a possible isocyanate residual to hydrolysis reactions, which can, in turn, provoke a serious food contamination. Some examples of multilayers structure obtained by lamination are shown in Table 6.2.

Another quite important source of PAA, as far as food contact materials are concerned, are azo colours which can be used in printing inks for plastic, paper and board, and largely used in black polyamide kitchen utensils (Trier et al. 2010).

6.2.3 Multi-injection Moulding

The same principle and issues of coextrusion, related to polymer compatibility at high temperature, can be applied to injection moulding technologies, largely used to obtain multilayers packages such as bottles, trays or closures.

A highlight of multi-injection moulding is the great variety of possible combinations; in fact, it allows producing layers from different thermoplastic polymers in one production step. This is the leading technology for plastic beer bottles and squeezable bottles for ketchup and similar products. Polyethylene terephthalate (PET) structural walls are sandwiched around a core of one or more layers containing higher oxygen and carbon dioxide barrier materials in these multilayer structures. Poly(m-xylyleneadipamide), also named PA/MXD 6, nanocomposites (see also Sect. 6.2.1), as passive barrier, and 'active' barrier systems, such as oxygen scavengers, are already in use for these products.

6.2.4 Coating

Coatings are recognised as powerful tools to improve many properties of packaging materials (Farris and Piergiovanni 2012). Coatings are intended to be general covering applied onto the surface of an object, defined as a substrate. In flexible packaging materials, coatings may be either external or sandwiched between two substrates. The thickness of such layers normally ranges from tenths of nanometers to few micrometres. Historically, the first coatings used on flexible packaging materials have been thin layers able to provide oxygen barrier, sealability and moisture resistance. However, coatings may provide various benefits to final materials such as better optical properties, especially ultraviolet absorption, higher or lower friction coefficient, scratch resistance and more or less wettability.

Polyvinylidene chloride (PVDC) copolymers, the oldest coatings used in packaging, are also the only organic lacquers provided in both organic solvent and aqueous dispersions. They are able to provide water vapour and oxygen barrier at once.

Ethylene vinyl alcohol copolymer is currently used as coating for critical applications in food and beverage packaging, due to its outstanding barrier property against oxygen. Polyvinyl alcohol (PVOH) coatings have the highest oxygen barrier; however, the high hydroxyl group content brings greater affinity to water, making PVOH coatings extremely sensitive to the surrounding relative humidity.

Acrylic polymers for coating formulations are available in various forms, though the emulsion form is the most widely used product. Nowadays, a great interest is related to the chance of using coating technology to increase the sustainability of packaging materials; i.e. to reduce the thickness of oil-derived conventional plastic films, by coating on them a thin layer of functional, high performing, bio-based material, etc. Two pertinent examples come from recent researches.

Cellulose nanocrystals (CNCs) obtained from cotton linters were used as coating on different substrates: PET, oriented polypropylene, oriented polyamide (OPA) and cellophane (Li et al. 2013). In comparison with the uncoated films, CNCs reduced friction coefficients preserving high transparency and low haze values; it also showed remarkable oxygen barrier properties, even better than most used barrier polymers. In addition, a mechanical abuse test (Gelbo flex test) was

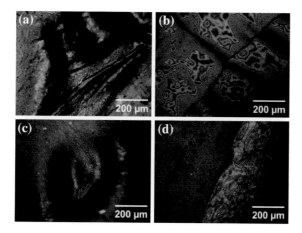

Fig. 6.3 The different strength of adhesion of cellulose nanocrystal (CNC) on four different films (**a** OPET, **b** OPP, **c** OPA, **d** cellophane), shown by the fracture patters after a GelboFlex test. Reproduced under permission from Li et al. (2015)

performed to understand the durability and strength of coatings. These last results demonstrated quite different interactions between CNCs and polymers; as shown in Fig. 6.3, fracture patterns were always different showing a better adhesion between CNCs and the most polar films (PET and OPA). Once again, the achievement of a successful coating, depends on the bonds at the interface, therefore, pretreatments are quite common in order to enhance chemical interactions. Besides, chemical primer (Wolf 2004), physical activation such as corona treatment (Sun et al. 1999) and flame treatment (Farris et al. 2010) are commonly used.

In another research (Farris et al. 2012), the development of high oxygen barrier coatings was achieved combining organic molecules (pullulan and other oil-derived polymers) with tetraethoxysilane, a metal alkoxide precursor of silica, as inorganic counterpart and intended to provide resistance to humidity. A schematic representation of expected reactions in sol–gel hybrid network formation is shown in Fig. 6.4. The development of such hybrid materials led to a new generation of coatings that are currently marketed under the OXAQUA® brand name.

6.2.5   Vacuum Metallisation

Packaging parts, films and sheets of plastic and paper can be coated with a metal for both aesthetic and functional purposes by means of a process called 'vacuum metallisation' (Sect. 3.2.2 about thermal properties of aluminum). Actually, aluminum is not the only metal that can be applied as a coating, even if by far the most important.

Optical density and oxygen barrier properties provided by various level of metallisation on a PET film are shown in Table 6.3. Basically, the metallisation

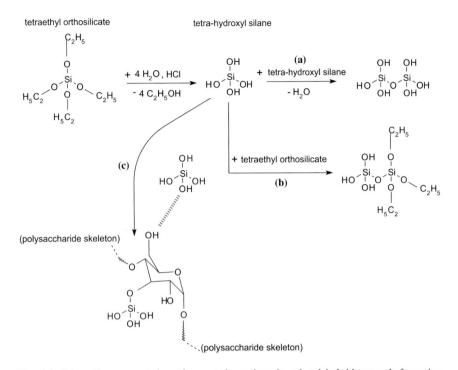

Fig. 6.4 Schematic representation of expected reactions in sol–gel hybrid network formation. Tetraethyl orthosilicate can be hydrolysed; this step requires low pH. The obtained tetra-hydroxyl silane can **a** react with the same molecule; the condensation can be observed. Alternatively, tetra-hydroxyl silane can react **b** with the original tetraethyl orthosilicate (alcohol condensation). Anyway, tetra-hydroxyl silane can be linked (Farris et al. 2012) with polysaccharide structures (covalent or hydrogen bonds). BKchem version 0.13.0, 2009 (http://bkchem.zirael.org/index.html) has been used for drawing these structures

Table 6.3 Optical density and oxygen barrier provided by various level of metallisation on a PET film

Metal layer (nm)	PO_2 (cm^3 d^{-1} bar^{-1} m^{-2})
0	45
12	1.55
29	0.77
36	0.62
39	0.26

The oxygen permeability, PO_2, has to be related to the following conditions: 25 μm, 23 °C, $\Delta RH = 0$ %

process requires the melting and the evaporation of metal that is fed inside a vacuum chamber as a thin wire, after which it condenses onto a web of cold substrate, passing above. Depending on the application, a plastic coating (mainly acrylic) may be applied after deposition to increase properties such as abrasion resistance and printability. If not only aesthetic properties are required, the very thin metal coating must be strictly homogeneous and continuous: in other words, it is well linked to the substrate. The adhesion of the metal on the plastic or cellulosic substrate, therefore, is the major point to be considered.

Various pretreatment methods to enhance adhesion are used and different theories and models describing the interaction between metals and polymers exist (Mark 1990; Jordan-Sweet 1990; De Bruyn et al. 2003). Roughening the substrate surface by grinding or chemical etching, for instance, introduces microporosities that enlarge the surface available for interaction, enhance metal atoms anchoring and promote nucleation sites. Other techniques to increase the metal adhesion to polymers are flame treatment, corona discharge and plasma activation. For these pretreatments, the mechanism of surface modification is the formation of a broad variety of oxygen containing functional groups, which better link the metal but may degrade the polymer surface too.

Apart from vacuum treatment, other techniques for materials metallisation such as 'arc' and 'flame spraying', 'electroless plating' and 'electroplating' do not find important applications in packaging.

6.2.6 Multilayered Cardboards Forming

Previously mentioned technologies are mostly related to multilayers structure, including plastic films. However, for their diffusion and relevance in food packaging applications, it is worthy to consider shortly also the structures completely or prevalently made with cellulose.

Many different paperboards (named 'multiply paperboards') are manufactured by creating various layers of pulps in the wet state, combining the advantages of different types of pulp in a single sheet of paperboard. Even if the same kind of pulp is used in all the layers, individual plies are treated and shaped independently to achieve the best possible quality. Multi-ply construction offers higher folding performance than single ply as a result of layering as it is shown in Fig. 6.5.

Fig. 6.5 Multi-ply structures offer higher folding performance as a result of plies layering

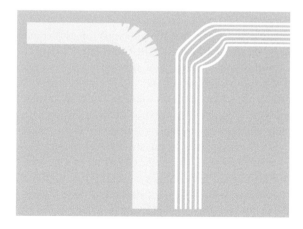

Because of the fibrous nature of the major constituents of pulps and entanglement possibilities, almost no problem of compatibility exists in these multilayers structures; however, glue or specific additives can be added to enhance the tightening of the plies.

6.3   Composites, Blend and Alloys

These possible routes to combine different materials are based on a mass mixture instead of layering different surfaces. When possible, they clearly offer technological advantages because a mixing operation is generally much simpler than lamination or coextrusion. On the contrary, issues related to the homogeneity and stability of these systems are definitely more serious.

6.3.1   Composites

A quite generic definition states that composite materials (also shortened to composites) are made from the interpenetration, i.e. an intimate mixture, of two or more constituent materials with physical or chemical properties significantly changed from the individual components. These materials generally remain in distinct domain within the finished structure, which appears, however, as a homogeneous material. The composite material may be stronger, lighter, less expensive or have more barrier properties than individual components. Typical composite materials include building materials (such as cements or concrete), metal matrix composites (at least, a metal in a different matrix), ceramic composites and reinforced plastics such as fibre-reinforced polymers.

In the packaging sector, major applications are about polymeric composites with fillers ranging from nano- to macroscale, generally in low percentage (less than 50 %), and addressed to many different kinds of materials enhancement. A growing importance, in particular, is related to nanocomposites as a new strategy to improve physical properties and functionality of plastic packaging materials (Reig et al. 2014; Arora and Padua 2010; Fabra et al. 2013).

A pertinent definition of nanomaterial is provided by a European resolution (European Commission 2011): 'a natural, incidental or manufactured material containing particles, in an unbound state or as an aggregate or as an agglomerate and where, for 50 % or more of the particles in the number size distribution, one or more external dimensions is in the size range 1–100 nm'.

Above the size definition, also the way of interaction among particles is relevant to the final application and to the chemistry of the composites. The terms 'agglomerate' and 'aggregate' are not always used properly, even if clear descriptions of different phenomena behind agglomeration and aggregation exist (European Commission 2011). Primary particles agglomerate to larger units by weak physical interactions, i.e.

by adhesion, leading to agglomerates. Agglomerates are, therefore, assemblies of particles joined together at the corners or edges, whose the total surface area is quite similar to the sum of specific surface areas of primary particles (Walter 2013). They are not fixed units but could change their size and shape, according to changes of temperature, pressure, pH value and viscosity of the surrounding medium. Aggregates develop when primary particles begin to form a common crystalline structure. From a physical–chemical point of view, the formation of aggregates is similar to the development of compact ceramic solids from several smaller particles (sintering process). Aggregates are an assembly of particles, aligned side by side (Walter 2013). Therefore, the total specific surface area is less than the sum of the surface areas of the primary particles. A sketch of the two phenomena is shown in Fig. 6.6.

The main driver of development of nanocomposites in food packaging is the need for higher barrier properties against gas, water vapour and aroma. Other important targets that could be reached by nanocomposites are functional barrier to unwanted specific migrants, improved thermal, optical, and mechanical properties and, finally, the development of active and intelligent devices. A possible

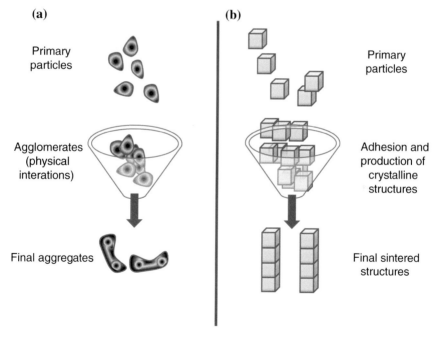

Fig. 6.6 Primary particles can agglomerate (**a**) to larger units without fixed dimensions: agglomerates could change their size and shape, according to changes of temperature, pressure, pH value and viscosity of the surrounding medium. Aggregates develop when primary particles begin to form a common crystalline structure. The formation of aggregates is similar to the development of compact ceramic solids from several smaller particles (sintering process). Should adhesion be the prevailing interaction (**b**), primary particles could aggregate with the production of crystalline structures (Walter 2013)

Table 6.4 Chemical families of fillers for plastic materials

Chemical family	Examples
Inorganics	
Oxides	Glass (fibres, spheres, hollow spheres, and flakes); magnesium oxide, antimony trioxide, silicon dioxide, aluminum oxide, titanium dioxide, zinc oxide
Hydroxides	Aluminum and magnesium hydroxides
Salts	Calcium carbonate, barium and calcium sulphates, phosphates, and hydrotalcite, etc.
Silicates	Talc, mica, kaolin, wollastonite, montmorillonite, feldspar, asbestos, etc.
Metals	Boron and steel
Carbon, graphite	Carbon fibres, graphite fibres and flakes, carbon nanotubes, and carbon black, grapheme, etc.
Organics	
Natural polymers	Cellulose fibres, wood flour and fibres, flax, cotton, sisal, starch, etc.
Synthetic polymers	Polyamide, polyester, aramid, polyvinyl alcohol fibres, etc.

classification of nanocomposites in flexible packaging materials refers to the nature of fillers that can be inorganic or organic and also bio-based (Table 6.4).

As inorganic fillers, montmorillonite and kaolinite clays are frequently used. They are two groups of aluminum-layered silicate minerals that have many other industrial uses, but have shown also good potential for improving barrier properties of polymeric materials. Between the aluminum silicate layers, there is a void region about 1 nm thick where positive ions like sodium, magnesium, calcium or lithium are located. This situation occurs because these clays are prone to cation exchange and to delayer by expansion phenomena of these void regions. Actually, three processes can take place in these corridors between silica layers:

- Hydrophobic modification; i.e. the cations may be exchanged with quaternary ammonium ions (e.g. cetyl-trialkyl-ammonium or cetyl-vinyl-dialkil-ammonium) changing a hydrophilic surface in a hydrophobic one that can definitely increase the compatibility with polymers
- Intercalation; i.e. a macromolecule is inserted in between the silica layers and linked, so the dimensions of interlayers remain fixed
- Exfoliation; i.e. a delaminating process wherein the interlayer thickness is greatly expanded leading to a disruption of the layers, spatially separated apart, creating a nanoscale dispersion in the matrix polymer. Clays exfoliation represents the nanomaterial; the achieved nanocomposite has very interesting barrier properties because nanoparticles act as physical hurdles to gas or vapour diffusion.

Graphene nanoplates are also very promising fillers (Uysal-Unalan et al. 2015). These carbon-based nanoparticles, at low loads (about 5 %), give improvements in barrier properties doubling that of the polymer matrix. Good compatibility between

Table 6.5 Particle morphology of fillers

Shape	Aspect ratio	Example
Cube	1	Feldspar and calcite
Sphere	1	Glass spheres, etc.
Block	1–4	Quartz, calcite, silica, barite, etc.
Plate	4–30	Kaolin, talc, hydrous alumina, etc.
Flake	50–200	Mica, graphite, montmorillonite nanoclays, etc.
Fibre	20–200	Wollastonite, glass fibres, carbon nanotubes, wood fibres, asbestos fibres, and carbon fibres, etc.

filler and polymer is essential; thus, further improvements could be expected from development of more compatible filler–polymer systems. Nanocomposites differ from conventional composite materials for the extremely high 'surface area/volume' (A/V) ratio and/or the very high aspect ratio (α). α is defined as the ratio of length over diameter for a fibre or the ratio of diameter over thickness for platelets and flakes. For example, spheres have α equal to the unity exhibiting minimal reinforcing capacity (Table 6.5).

The large increase of available surface means that a small amount of nanofiller can have significant effects on macroscale properties (Xanthos 2005). Therefore, the mass fraction of the nanoparticles (weight %) can remain very low in the range from 0.5 to 5 %.

In mechanical terms, high α and A/V values correspond to a great reinforcing function, which is also a very attractive target for packaging materials. High A/V ratio can speed up thermodynamic processes that minimise free energy: thus, nano-composite reacts much faster because more surface is available to react. Figure 6.7 shows (Fischer 2003; Gacitua et al. 2005; McCrum et al. 1997; Xanthos 2005) that maximising A/V and particle–matrix interaction through the interface requires $\alpha \gg 1$ for fibres (on the right) and $1/\alpha \ll 1$ for platelets (on the left).

Many polymer properties, very relevant to packaging, are significantly affected near the nanofiller. The degree of thermoset cure, polymer chain mobility and chain conformation or crystallinity can all vary significantly and continuously from the interface with nanoparticles into the bulk of the matrix (Ajayan et al. 2006).

With concern to opportunities provided by bio-based materials, it should be underlined that inorganic nanoclays have been extensively studied as possible reinforcing agents and functional fillers of bio-based polymers (Mascheroni et al. 2010). A great interest exists also about the chance of improving mechanical properties of common polymers, using bio-based nanoparticles.

In particular, cellulose nanoparticles have been investigated as possible reinforcing filler of various polymers such as polylactic acid, polystyrene and low-density polyethylene (Miao and Hamad 2013). The main issue is related to the poor dispersibility of nanocellulose inside the polymeric matrix, because of its hydrophilic nature and its agglomeration caused by strong interchain hydrogen bonds (Moon et al. 2011). Chemical changes, mainly esterification, have been

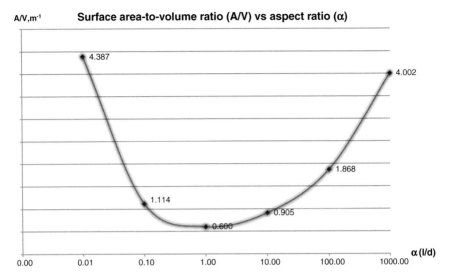

Fig. 6.7 A simplified representation of the relationship between the 'surface area/volume' (A/V) ratio and aspect ratio (α) values, for cylindrical particles with constant volume (Fischer 2003; Gacitua et al. 2005; McCrum et al. 1997; Xanthos 2005)

extensively used to solve these problems. Moreover, it is worthy to mention a quite new class of composites based on cellulosic materials only, called 'all-cellulose composites' (ACC). These advanced materials are not always based on nanocellulose, but they have been proposed and produced using various cellulosic fibres (Li et al. 2015).

Main routes used for ACC preparation are an impregnation of cellulose matrix into cellulose fibres and a selective dissolution where cellulose external fibres are partially dissolved to form a matrix phase that bonds fibres together. The last method leads to the highest ever reported mechanical properties for a natural fibre-reinforced composite (Eichhorn et al. 2010), because of the dissolution of fibre outer layers which mainly consist of amorphous cellulose, while the remaining core consists of highly oriented and crystalline regions (Lu et al. 2003).

6.3.2   *Polymer Blends and Alloys*

Polymer blends are macroscopically (on scales which are several times the wavelengths of visible light) a homogeneous mixture of two or more different polymeric species. No account is taken of the miscibility or immiscibility of the constituent macromolecules, i.e. no assumption is made regarding the number of phase domains present. In fact, miscibility is the capability of a mixture to form a single phase over certain ranges of temperature, pressure and composition. Whereas, immiscibility is the inability of a mixture to form a single phase. This property may be limited to certain ranges of temperature, pressure and composition; it depends on chemical structures, molar mass distributions and molecular architectures of involved components (Utracki and Wilkie 2014).

According to the International Union of Pure and Applied Chemistry (IUPAC), the term 'polymer alloy' refers to a polymeric material, exhibiting macroscopically uniform physical properties. It includes compatible polymer blends (immiscible polymer blend that exhibits macroscopically uniform physical properties due to sufficiently strong interactions between the component polymers), monophase polymer blends (miscible) or multiphase copolymers (Alemán et al. 2007). In this definition, incompatible polymer blends are excluded. In other words, all polymer alloys are blends, but not all polymer blends are alloys.

Because of the complexity and risk of misunderstanding, IUPAC discourages the use of the term 'polymer alloy' for a polymer blend. Should the blend be made of two immiscible polymers, two glass transition temperatures would be observed. On the other hand, should the blend be a single-phase structure (miscible), one glass transition temperature would be observed.

Packaging applications of polymer blends and alloys in packaging are many and diverse; they refer to films, container, closures and shipping containers. Compatibilised polymer alloys have been developed in order to enhance process-ability under thermoforming conditions and to give the moulded articles produced superior gloss, surface hardness, strength and high heat distortion. Broad applications of blend and alloys are related to the manufacturing of adhesives for lamination and to the development of barrier materials (Finlayson 1994). A blend of the copolymer PET/ethylene-methacrylic acid copolymer (EMAA) was found to have high barrier properties against hydrocarbon and other solvents. A polyamide 6/MXD-6 blend has gas permeability comparable to PVDC. A PVC/styrene maleic anhydride blend increases the thermal stability till at high temperature (30' at 110 ° C) making feasible a microwaveable hot-fill food packaging.

References

Ajayan PM, Schadler LS, Braun PV (2006) Nanocomposite science and technology. Wiley, New York

Alemán JV, Chadwick AV, He J, Hess M, Horie K, Jones RG, Kratochvíl P, Meisel I, Mita I, Moad G, Penczek S, Stepto RFT (2007) Definitions of terms relating to the structure and processing of sols, gels, networks, and inorganic-organic hybrid materials (IUPAC Recommendations 2007). Pure Appl Chem 79(10):1801–1829. doi:10.1351/pac200779101801

Arora A, Padua GW (2010) Review: nanocomposites in food packaging. J Food Sci 75(1): R43–R49. doi:10.1111/j.1750-3841.2009.01456.x

Bishop CA, Mount EM III (2010) Vacuum metallizing for flexible packaging. In: Wagner JR (ed) Multilayer flexible packaging. William Andrew Publishing, Boston

De Bruyn K, Van Stappen M, De Deurwaerder H, Rouxhet L, Celis JP (2003) Study of pretreatment methods for vacuum metallization of plastics. Surf Coat Technol 163–164:710–715. doi:http://dx.doi.org/10.1016/S0257-8972(02)00684-9

de Fátima Poças M, Hogg T (2007) Exposure assessment of chemicals from packaging materials in foods: a review. Trends Food Sci Technol 18(4):219–230. doi:http://dx.doi.org/10.1016/j.tifs. 2006.12.008

Eichhorn SJ, Dufresne A, Aranguren M, Marcovich NE, Capadona JR, Rowan SJ, Weder C, Thielemans W, Roman M, Renneckar S, Gindl W, Veigel S, Keckes J, Yano H, Abe K, Nogi M, Nakagaito AN, Mangalam A, Simonsen J, Benight AS, Bismarck A, Berglund LA, Peijs T (2010) Review: current international research into cellulose nanofibres and nanocomposites. J Mater Sci 45(1):1–33. doi:10.1007/s10853-009-3874-0

European Commission (2011) Commission Recommendation of 18 October 2011 on the definition of nanomaterial. Off J Eur Union L275:38–40. http://eur-lex.europa.eu/legal-content/EN/ ALL/?uri=CELEX:32011H0696. Accessed 18 May 2015

Fabra MJ, Busolo MA, Lopez-Rubio A, Lagaron JM (2013) Nanostructured biolayers in food packaging. Trends Food Sci Technol 31(1):79–87. doi:http://dx.doi.org/10.1016/j.tifs.2013.01. 004

Farris S, Piergiovanni L (2012) Emerging coating technologies for food and beverage packaging materials. In: Yam KL, Lee DS (eds) Emerging food packaging technologies. Woodhead Publishing Ltd, England

Farris S, Pozzoli S, Biagioni P, Duó L, Mancinelli S, Piergiovanni L (2010) The fundamentals of flame treatment for the surface activation of polyolefin polymers—a review. Polym 51 (16):3591–3605. doi:10.1016/j.polymer.2010.05.036

Farris S, Introzzi L, Fuentes-Alventosa JM, Santo N, Rocca R, Piergiovanni L (2012) Self-assembled pullulan-silica oxygen barrier hybrid coatings for food packaging applications. J Agric Food Chem 60(3):782–790. doi:10.1021/Jf204033d

Finlayson K (1994) Advances in polymer blends and alloys technology, vol V. Technomic Publishing Company Inc, Lancaster

Fischer H (2003) Polymer nanocomposites: from fundamental research to specific applications. Mater Sci Eng C 23(6):763–772. doi:10.1016/j.msec.2003.09.148

Franz R, Störmer A (2008) Migration of plastic constituents. In: Piringer OG, Baner AL (eds) Plastic packaging. Wiley-VCH Verlag GmbH & Co. KGaA, Weinheim. doi:10.1002/ 9783527621422.ch11

Franz R, Kluge S, Lindner A, Piringer O (1990) Cause of catty odour formation in packaged food. Packag Technol Sci 3(2):89–95. doi:10.1002/pts.2770030206

Gacitua W, Ballerini A, Zhang J (2005) Polymer nanocomposites: synthetic and natural fillers a review. Maderas Cienc Tecnol 7(3):159–178. doi:10.4067/S0718-221X2005000300002

Grönman K, Soukka R, Järvi-Kääriäinen T, Katajajuuri J-M, Kuisma M, Koivupuro H-K, Ollila M, Pitkänen M, Miettinen O, Silvenius F, Thun R, Wessman H, Linnanen L (2013) Framework for sustainable food packaging design. Packag Technol Sci 26(4):187–200. doi:10. 1002/pts.1971

Gutoff EB, Cohen ED (2010) Water- and solvent-based coating technology. In: Wagner JR (ed) Multilayer Flexible Packaging. William Andrew Publishing, Boston

Jordan-Sweet JL (1990) Using near-edge soft X-ray absorption spectroscopy to study organic polymers and metal-polymer interactions. In: Sacher E, Pireaux JJ, Kowalczyk SP (eds) Metallization of polymers, ACS Symp Ser, vol 440, pp 242–264. American Chemical Society, Columbus. doi:10.1021/bk-1990-0440.ch018

Li F, Biagioni P, Bollani M, Maccagnan A, Piergiovanni L (2013) Multi-functional coating of cellulose nanocrystals for flexible packaging applications. Cellul 20(5):2491–2504. doi:10. 1007/s10570-013-0015-3

Li F, Mascheroni E, Piergiovanni L (2015) The potential of nanocellulose in the packaging field: a review. Packag Technol Sci 28(6):475–564. doi:10.1002/pts.2121

Lu X, Zhang MQ, Rong MZ, Shi G, Yang GC (2003) Self-reinforced melt processable composites of sisal. Compos Sci Technol 63(2):177–186. doi:10.1016/S0266-3538(02)00204-X

Mark PA (1990) Reactions of metal atoms with monomers and polymers. In: Sacher E, Pireaux JJ, Kowalczyk SP (eds) Metallization of polymers, ACS Symp Ser, vol 440, pp 242–264. American Chemical Society, Columbus. doi:10.1021/bk-1990-0440.ch018

Mascheroni E, Chalier P, Gontard N, Gastaldi E (2010) Designing of a wheat gluten/montmorillonite based system as carvacrol carrier: rheological and structural properties. Food Hydrocoll 24(4):406–413. doi:10.1016/j.foodhyd.2009.11.007

McCrum NG, Buckley CP, Bucknall CB (1997) Principles of Polymer Engineering, 2nd edn. Oxford University Press, New York, pp 242–245

Miao C, Hamad W (2013) Cellulose reinforced polymer composites and nanocomposites: a critical review. Cellul 20(5):2221–2262. doi:10.1007/s10570-013-0007-3

Moon RJ, Martini A, Nairn J, Simonsen J, Youngblood J (2011) Cellulose nanomaterials review: structure, properties and nanocomposites. Chem Soc Rev 40:3941–3994. doi:10.1039/c0cs00108b

Mount E III (2010) Coextrusion equipment for multilayer flat films and sheets. In: Wagner JR (ed) Multilayer flexible packaging. William Andrew Publishing, Boston, pp 75–95

Reig CS, Lopez AD, Ramos MH, Ballester VAC (2014) Nanomaterials: a map for their selection in food packaging applications. Packag Technol Sci 27(11):839–866. doi:10.1002/pts.2076

Silvenius F, Grönman K, Katajajuuri J-M, Soukka R, Koivupuro H-K, Virtanen Y (2014) The role of household food waste in comparing environmental impacts of packaging alternatives. Packag Technol Sci 27(4):277–292. doi:10.1002/pts.2032

Sun C, Zhang D, Wadsworth LC (1999) Corona treatment of polyolefin films—a review. Adv Polymer Technol 18(2):171–180. doi:10.1002/(SICI)1098-2329(199922)18:2<171:AID-ADV6>3.0.CO;2-8

Trier X, Okholm B, Foverskov A, Binderup ML, Petersen JH (2010) Primary aromatic amines (PAAs) in black nylon and other food-contact materials, 2004–2009. Food Addit Contam Part A 27(9):1325–1335. doi:10.1080/19440049.2010.487500

Utracki LA, Wilkie CA (2014) Polymer blends handbook. Springer Reference. Springer Science +Business Media B.V, Dordrecht

Uysal Ünalan IU, Wan C, Trabattoni S, Piergiovanni L, Farris S (2015) Polysaccharide-assisted rapid exfoliation of graphite platelets into high quality water-dispersible graphene sheets. RSC Adv 5(34):26482–26490. doi:10.1039/C4RA16947F

Wagner JR Jr (2010) Blown film, cast film and lamination processes. In: Wagner JR (ed) Multilayer flexible packaging. William Andrew Publishing, Boston

Walter D (2013) Primary particles–agglomerates–aggregates. Nanomaterials. Wiley-VCH Verlag GmbH & Co. KGaA, Weinheim, pp 9–24

Wikström F, Williams H (2010) Potential environmental gains from reducing food losses through development of new packaging—a life-cycle model. Packag Technol Sci 23(7):403–411. doi:10.1002/pts.906

Wolf AR (2004) Surface activation systems for optimizing adhesion to polymers. In: Conference Proceedings of the ANTEC Conference 2004. Society of Plastics Engineers, Bethel

Xanthos M (2005) Polymers and polymer composites. In: Xanthos M (ed) Functional fillers for plastics. Wiley-VCH Verlag GmbH & Co. KGaA, Weinheim, pp 1–16

Chapter 7
Chemical Features of Food Packaging Materials

Abstract Chemistry is not only important in the production of packaging materials. Important reactions may take place or must occur during practical uses, when packages are filled with food and beverages and, after their use, addressed to recycling processes. For various reasons, these chemical changes can be very important; as a result, the most relevant ones of these modifications—corrosion, cracking, fractures, weathering, etc.—should be shortly discussed. Corrosion is usually referred to metals and, more rarely, to concrete, polymers and glasses. This complex phenomenon depends on different variables. Also, biodegradation and compostability have to be discussed when speaking of food packaging materials. Chemical resistance can be indirectly described in terms of stability to oxidation, resistance to corrosion and other performances. In addition, peculiar abuse tests are available when speaking of the resistance of materials under the combined effects of a stress and aggressive environmental. Consequently, modifications of weight, dimensions, mechanical properties and visual appearance are evaluated in order to express a rate of chemical resistance.

Keywords Abuse test · Biodegradation · Compostability · Corrosion · Cracking · Etching · Fracture · Leaching · Recalcitrance · Weathering

Abbreviations

ESC Environmental stress cracking
M   Metal
MW   Molecular weight
TFS Tin-free steel

7.1 Food Packaging Materials: Chemical Features

Chemistry is not only important in the production of packaging materials. In fact, important reactions may take place or must occur during practical uses, when packages are filled with food and beverages (possibly processed with them) and,

© The Author(s) 2016
L. Piergiovanni and S. Limbo, *Food Packaging Materials*,
Chemistry of Foods, DOI 10.1007/978-3-319-24732-8_7

after their use, addressed to recycling processes. For various reasons, these chemical changes can be very important; as a result, the most relevant ones of these modifications should be shortly presented in conclusion.

7.2 Corrosion

Corrosion is generally defined as the phenomenon leading to a gradual destruction of whatever material that is interacting with environment or contact media components. It is usually referred to metals and, more rarely, to concrete, polymers and glasses. As far as packaging materials are concerned, glass corrosion is worth to be considered, even if it much less common and significant.

Glass corrosion goes through two distinct steps which may occur consecutively or separately (Clark et al. 1979). The first one is due to water contact when an ion exchange occurs between sodium ions from glass surfaces and hydrogen ions from water solution. Consequently, the effective surface area in contact with the solution is increased and the pH may increase. These two phenomena can promote the second step, which corresponds to leaching of alkali ions from the glass, leaving a silica-rich layer on the surface. This second stage of glass corrosion is a much more relevant destruction process of the glass surface, even if very limited in real cases of food packaging.

Actually, glass is resistant to most acids but highly susceptible to alkaline solutions, especially at pH greater than 9.0, which are definitely uncommon in food and beverages but not in detergents used for refillable bottles. Repeated cycles of washing and refilling glass containers can actually lead to a loss in transparency: these phenomena are called glass corrosion.

In the most common sense, corrosion means metal rusting. The formation of iron oxides is the most known, but not unique phenomenon, of the electrochemical oxidation of metals. As glass corrosion, also metal corrosion is a diffusion-controlled process: it occurs on exposed surfaces. For this reason, every technology able to reduce the exposed surface, such as passivation and coating, is so important in packaging applications. The control of corrosion is of great concern to packaging manufacturers, as well as to food processors because products of metal corrosion may affect the quality of packaged foods and the hermetic integrity of the packages (Harlow and Wei 1998, 2002).

When a metal is in a moist environment or in contact with aqueous solution, the metal surface acts as an electrode and the contained food may act as an electrolytic solution transferring the electric current created by electrons transfer. When the metal surface corrodes, in fact, the metal (M) oxidises to its cationic form (M^{n+}) and leaves the generated electrons on the surface.

$$M \rightarrow M^{n+} + ne^-$$ (7.1)

Some components in the food, receiving the generated electrons, will become reduced accordingly. The electrode with oxidation reaction is called anode (the metal) whereas the electrode with reduction reaction (food component) is called cathode. Each metal has a different tendency in acting as an electrode, explained by its thermodynamics (Gibbs free energy) that is generally expressed by standard reduction potential (Eo) with reference to hydrogen electrode standardised to potential zero (Table 7.1). Metals with higher positive Eo values show stability in contact with an aqueous medium because they have a tendency to exist as a reduced form.

Because electrode reactions should always be coupled, i.e. oxidation and reduction reactions have to occur contemporary, a metal with higher Eo might work as a cathode (having reduction reaction), while another one, with lower Eo, would work as an anode (oxidation, as reverse direction of reactions in the table). In addition, temperature and pH values can strongly influence the rate and the extent of corrosion phenomena; in fact, passivation films on some metallic surface are generally able to stop the anodic oxidation and the cathodic reduction only within defined pH ranges.

Various and different corrosion events may actually occur in real food packaging applications. Since corrosion phenomena depend on several factors, each one being a function of several variables, their complete description remains beyond the scope of this book; only few examples, referring to important real cases, are presented in this chapter.

The majority of tinplate cans for food packaging applications are used as internally lacquered for protecting steel plate against corrosion; however, some packaged foods, such as tomato products, peaches, pineapple, citrus juices and mushrooms, are successfully packed in not lacquered, high-tin-coating (>10 g m^{-2}) tinplate cans (Turner 1991). With concern to corrosion behaviour, tin acts as anode, while the cathode would be represented by the reduction of dissolved oxygen. In

Table 7.1 Standard reduction potential (Eo) for some selected electrodes

Electrode	Standard reduction potential (V)	
$Au^{2+} + 2\,e^- \rightarrow Au$	+1.50	
$1/2\,O_2 + 2\,H^+ + 2\,e^- \rightarrow H_2O$	+1.23	+0.81 at pH = 7
$Ag^+ + e^- \rightarrow Ag$	+0.80	
$Fe^{3+} + e^- \rightarrow Fe^{2+}$	+0.77	
$1/2\,O_2 + H_2O + 2\,e^- \rightarrow 2\,OH^-$	+0.40	+0.81 at pH = 7
$Cu^{2+} + 2\,e^- \rightarrow Cu$	+0.34	
$2\,H^+ + 2\,e^- \rightarrow H_2$	+0.00 (reference)	
$Pb^{2+} + 2\,e^- \rightarrow Pb$	−0.13	
$Sn^{2+} + 2\,e^- \rightarrow Sn$	−0.14	
$Ni^{2+} + 2\,e^- \rightarrow Ni$	−0.25	
$Fe^{2+} + 2\,e^- \rightarrow Fe$	−0.44	
$Cr^{3+} + 3\,e^- \rightarrow Cr$	−0.74	
$Al^{3+} + 3\,e^- \rightarrow Al$	−1.66	

these situations, oxygen is usefully consumed after a short time of packaging due to their acidic content. Cathodic reactions occur at reduced rate, resulting in controlled and limited detinning that may become critical only after 1.5–2 years at 25 °C (Charbonneau 1997). Whereas the tin coating is not enough to protect against corrosion, or too much oxygen is inside the container, iron dissolution may take place and lead to hydrogen production. The evolved gas into the headspace would even cause cans to swell and/or to lead to pitting, i.e. small perforation and leaking of the product.

The breakdown of food proteins containing sulphur amino acids, such as cysteine, cystine and methionine, can lead in some instances to accelerated corrosion phenomena. In canned food products, after heat processing, this behaviour may lead to unpleasant dark staining of tinplate surfaces and sensorial defects of preserved foods. Sulphide ions can react with tin and iron to produce tin or iron sulphide, which cause visible staining defects on the metal surface without toxic risks for consumers. Obviously, the external surface of tinplate may also corrode leading to localised rust or stains; in particular, an excessive use of chlorine in cooling water, as well as long-time exposure to wet environment, may cause external corrosion of tinplate.

Corrosion of tin-free steel (TFS) plates is less frequent, due to the very good resistance against rusting and corrosion (Robertson 1993; Charbonneau 1997) of chromium oxides and the excellent adhesion of protective lacquering. However, TFS cans are also prone to filiform corrosion and possible perforations, particularly if the passivation layer is not continuous on the surface (Morita and Yoshida 1994).

As already mentioned in Sect. 3.2, aluminum oxide (Al_2O_3) is formed as passivation layer on the metal surface. However, it may dissolve under acidic or alkaline conditions or be removed by some complexing ligands (Robertson 1993) such as citric, malic and phosphoric acid, sulphites or anthocyanin pigments, leading to the corrosion of aluminum cans.

Moreover, aluminum cans are prone to be corroded by chloride ions in food products. Chlorides can cause typical perforation (pitting) of the can body, particularly if associated to high temperature, low pH values and high oxygen concentration conditions (Piergiovanni et al. 1990). External corrosion of aluminum packages occurs rarely: it is favoured by mechanical stresses and wet or dirty conditions of storage.

Stainless steels used in food packaging applications are rarely subject to corrosion phenomena. These reactions can be driven only by very strong acidic concentration and after an unlikely local loss of passivation film, which may lead to active spots behaving as a galvanic cell. Pitting and crevice formation are steel corrosion phenomena occurring by this mechanism (Pardo et al. 2000).

If a metal surface stays in humid conditions for a long time, it may be colonised by microorganisms able to form so-called 'biofilms'. Their colonies are held together by polymeric substances (e.g. exopolysaccharides and lipopolysaccharides) produced by the cells themselves. These large molecules provide adhesion and stability to the biofilm and deeply change local chemical composition.

Microbial biofilms cause several problems, not only from a hygienic point of view, because they can particularly contribute to corrosion (Kumar and Anand 1998; Little et al. 2007). The microbiologically induced corrosion is a very dangerous form of attack on metallic materials that can cause damages to metals in contact with water supply systems, as well as in cooling circuits of processing plants, but rarely in food packaging applications.

7.3   Degradability

For a long time, the possible degradation of packaging objects, especially food packaging materials, has been considered as a critical aspect and strictly avoided, looking for materials with high inertia and low reactivity. The issues of waste management and packaging sustainability changed dramatically the point of view; nowadays, it became important to have biodegradable packaging materials with the ability of evaluating biodegradability accurately.

According to the International Union of Pure and Applied Chemistry, biodegradability is the 'capability of being degraded by biological activity' (Horie et al. 2004). This definition excludes abiotic enzymatic processes, i.e. the in vitro activity of isolated enzymes, saying nothing about final products of the degradation. In fact biodegradation does not necessarily involve mineralisation, i.e. the conversion of carbon, nitrogen, sulphur and phosphorous content to simple inorganic products but, ineludibly, it refers to organic materials only.

Generally speaking, all biosynthetic materials (such as cellulose or polyhydroxyalkanoate) should biodegrade while synthetic materials cannot be able to exhibit this behaviour. However, several exceptions are known (and already stated) due to different reasons.

Recalcitrance is called the tendency of some molecules to escape biodegradation. This behaviour might be due to the molecular weight (MW): in fact a MW equal to 500 Da is generally considered the cut-off to the ability of living organisms to metabolise substances. Other possible reasons for recalcitrance are the presence of molecules incompatible with enzymatic attack, hydrophobicity and the presence of chemical residuals unfavourable for bacterial growth (Alexander 1965).

According to many international standards, biodegradation is evaluated measuring the amount of inorganic carbon dioxide produced by a selected population of microorganisms from the inoculated material. Some misunderstandings often occur about the following two terms: 'biodegradable' and 'compostable'. The latter is the ability to undergo biological decomposition in a compost site, in specific conditions and consistent with known compostable materials. Actually, the biological decomposition depends on various factors of the environmental conditions such as moisture, temperature and others variables.

Definitely, the definition of compostability seems a more clear and useful property, relying on specific conditions; in accordance with the European harmonised EN

13432 norm, a material is considered compostable if at least 90 % of it biodegrades in a specified test within 6 months (Kijchavengkul and Auras 2008).

Biodegradation and compostability, as already stated, refer to organic materials but, more in general, we can talk about 'degradability' of whatever material, including glasses, metals and oil based polymers. This discussion, however, deals with various different processes and phenomena which are better represented in terms of chemical resistance of packaging materials.

7.4   Chemical Resistance

The ability of solid materials to resist damages by chemical reactivity or solvent action is named 'chemical resistance' or also 'chemical compatibility'. The property refers to an overall capacity of a material to maintain its fundamental characteristics when exposed to some chemically aggressive substance; it may be very important or even crucial for all packaging materials during manufacturing, using, recycling and wasting (ASTM 2014). 'Etching', 'leaching' and 'weathering' are also general terms quite often used to indicate materials degradation and chemical resistance tests. The first two terms are related to possible matter removal from the surfaces of packaging materials by dissolution or scraping, while weathering is the chemical decomposition or physical damage of a material on exposure to different, aggressive atmospheres. To evaluate these various material behaviours, many tests have been developed by different organisations linked to material producers or users.

In general, these chemical performances are measured by means of so-called 'abuse tests', which means that standardised sample materials are exposed in standardised contact conditions to a chemical substance. The changes of weight (due to absorption or leaching), dimension (due to absorption or interaction), mechanical properties and appearance (due to possible chemical transformations) are evaluated subjectively or objectively measured after time, in order to express a rate of chemical resistance.

Other relevant examples of chemical performances, important to food packaging materials, include stability to oxidation, combustion behaviour, resistance to corrosion, oil or grease penetration. Both for metal and plastic materials, a special type of failure tests under environmental effects are known and commonly evaluated.

'Environmental Stress Fracture' (for metals) and 'Environmental Stress Cracking' (also named ESC, for plastics) describe unexpected brittle failure of samples exposed to chemicals possibly used in cleaning or lubrication. The combined effects of a stress and aggressive environmental tend to accelerate and pro mote a cracking phenomenon which, each one alone, would not be enough to cause (Ezrin and Lavigne 2007).

These materials features are seldom defined clearly and associated with accurately measurable phenomena. Even if they definitely belong to a domain of empirical evaluation, one more time they underline the importance of controlling and investigating the chemistry of packaging materials.

References

Alexander M (1965) Biodegradation: problems of molecular recalcitrance and microbial fallibility. Adv Appl Microbiol 7:35–80. doi:10.1016/S0065-2164(08)70383-6

ASTM (2014) Active Standard ASTM D543-14—Standard practices for evaluating the resistance of plastics to chemical reagents, ASTM Volume 08.01 Plastics (I): C1147 D3159. ASTM International, West Conshohocken. doi:10.1520/D0543-14

Charbonneau JE (1997) Recent case histories of food product-metal container interactions using scanning electron microscopy-X-ray microanalysis. Scan 19(7):512–518. doi:10.1002/sca.4950190710

Clark DE, Pantano Jr CG, Hench LL (1979) Corrosion of glass. Glass Industry, Books for Industry and The Glass Industry, Division of Magazines for Industry, Inc. New York

Ezrin M, Lavigne G (2007) Unexpected and unusual failures of polymeric materials. Eng Fail Anal 14(6):1153–1165. doi:10.1016/j.engfailanal.2006.11.048

Harlow D, Wei R (1998) A probability model for the growth of corrosion pits in aluminum alloys induced by constituent particles. Eng Fract Mech 59(3):305–325. doi:10.1016/S0013-7944(97)00127-6

Harlow DG, Wei RP (2002) A critical comparison between mechanistically based probability and statistically based modeling for materials aging. Mater Sci Eng A 323(1–2):278–284. doi:10.1016/S0921-5093(01)01370-3

Horie K, Barón M, Fox RB, He J, Hess M, Kahovec J, Kitayama T, Kubisa P, Maréchal E, Mormann W, Stepto RFT, Tabak D, Vohlídal J, Wilks ES, Work WJ (2004) Definitions of terms relating to reactions of polymers and to functional polymeric materials (IUPAC Recommendations 2003). Pure Appl Chem 76(4):889–906. doi:10.1351/pac200476040889

Kijchavengkul T, Auras R (2008) Compostability of polymers. Polym Int 57(6):793–804. doi:10.1002/pi.2420

Kumar CG, Anand S (1998) Significance of microbial biofilms in food industry: a review. Int J Food Microbiol 42(1–2):9–27. doi:10.1016/S0168-1605(98)00060-9

Little BJ, Mansfeld FB, Arps PJ, Earthman JC (2007) Microbiologically influenced corrosion. Wiley-VCH Verlag GmbH & Co. KGaA, Weinheim. doi:10.1002/9783527610426.bard040603

Morita J, Yoshida M (1994) Effects of free tin on filiform corrosion behavior of lightly tin-coated steel. Corros 50(1):11–19. doi:10.5006/1.3293489

Pardo A, Otero E, Merino M, López M, Utrilla M, Moreno F (2000) Influence of pH and chloride concentration on the pitting and crevice corrosion behavior of high-alloy stainless steels. Corros 56(4):411–418. doi:10.5006/1.3280545

Piergiovanni L, Fava P, Ciappellano S, Testolin G (1990) Modelling acidic corrosion of aluminium foil in contact with foods. Packag Technol Sci 3(4):195–201. doi:10.1002/pts.2770030404

Robertson GL (1993) Food packaging: principles and practice. Marcel Dekker, New York, pp 173–231

Turner T (1991) Packaging of heat preserved foods in metal containers. In: Rees JAG, Bettison J (eds) Processing and packaging heat preserved foods. Springer, New York, p 92

Printed in the United States
By Bookmasters